||||||||||||||||||||||||||||||||||
D0645903

HERE ARE THE FACTS:

- No individual diagnosed as having AIDS before 1981 is alive today.

- The average life expectancy of an AIDS patient after his or her diagnosis is 18 months.

- There are at least one million Americans currently infected with the AIDS virus.

- More than 90% of the Americans who are now infected with the AIDS virus are unaware of their infection.

- Blood screening plans for 1985 will identify fewer than 1% of the symptomless carriers.

...BUT YOU CAN *STILL* PROTECT YOURSELF AND YOUR FAMILY.

THE AIDS EPIDEMIC presents all the known facts about this dread disease, answers hundreds of your pressing questions, and offers a clear, sane summons to personal preservation and social responsibility in the face of the greatest threat to public health in America today.

ABOUT THE AUTHORS

James I. Slaff, M.D., graduated from Yale University in 1975 and the University of Virginia Medical School in 1979. He received his postgraduate training in Internal Medicine and Gastroenterology at the University of Florida. Currently Dr. Slaff is a Medical Investigator at the National Institutes of Health in Bethesda, Maryland. He lives in Maryland with his wife and their daughter.

A writer and social scientist, John K. Brubaker graduated from Yale University in 1976. He currently resides in Sound Beach, on Long Island, New York.

ATTENTION: SCHOOLS AND CORPORATIONS

WARNER books are available at quantity discounts with bulk purchase for educational, business, or sales promotional use. For information, please write: SPECIAL SALES DEPARTMENT, WARNER BOOKS, 666 FIFTH AVENUE, NEW YORK, N.Y. 10103.

ARE THERE WARNER BOOKS
YOU WANT BUT CANNOT FIND IN YOUR LOCAL STORES?

You can get any WARNER BOOKS title in print. Simply send title and retail price, plus 50¢ per order and 50¢ per copy to cover mailing and handling costs for each book desired. New York State and California residents add applicable sales tax. Enclose check or money order only, no cash please, to: WARNER BOOKS, P.O. BOX 690, NEW YORK, N.Y. 10019

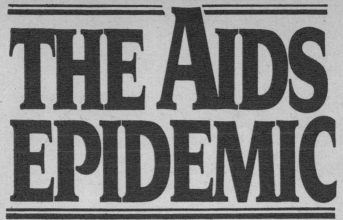

THE AIDS EPIDEMIC

How You Can Protect Yourself and Your Family— Why You Must

JAMES I. SLAFF, M.D.,
and JOHN K. BRUBAKER

WARNER BOOKS

A Warner Communications Company

THE AIDS EPIDEMIC: *How You Can Protect Yourself and Your Family—Why You Must* was written by Dr. James I. Slaff in his private capacity. No official support or endorsement by the National Institutes of Health is intended or should be inferred.

WARNER BOOKS EDITION

Copyright © 1985 by James I. Slaff and John K. Brubaker
All rights reserved.

Warner Books, Inc.
666 Fifth Avenue
New York, N.Y. 10103

A Warner Communications Company

Printed in the United States of America

First Printing: December, 1985

10 9 8 7 6 5 4 3 2 1

To my grandfather, Frank Slaff
January 5, 1897–April 13, 1979

J.I.S.

To my father, John St. Cyr Brubaker
July 12, 1924–May 5, 1985

J.K.B.

ACKNOWLEDGMENTS

We would like to gratefully acknowledge those who made valuable contributions to this project:

Mario Sartori for his sensitivity and editorial input. Patti Breitman for her boundless enthusiasm and support, and to them both for being such a delight to work with. And also to the staff at Warner Books for demonstrating extraordinary vision and commitment in making this work so rapidly available.

Jonathan Slaff contributed his research skill, editorial advice, and many long weekends. He is responsible for much of Chapter 4.

Don Gastwirth, our agent, unstintingly gave his professional acumen, persistent spirit, and generous encouragement from the first days.

Jan Wilhite of Gainesville, Florida, and Aggie Griffin of Datatype Associates in Lanham, Maryland, demonstrated word processing expertise and personal grace under constant pressure in taking the manuscript from the roughest draft to its final form. Alan Hall Printing of Lanham provided timely copying.

Thanks to Al Davis for his consistent strategic and tactical brilliance—given over a period of many years.

Dr. Zaki Salahuddin and Dr. Rodger Bell provided valued scientific assistance.

Dan Case, Mike Colucci, Stefana Matarazza, and Bobby Welch gave valued special knowledge.

Thanks to those who, for personal reasons, wish to maintain relative anonymity—S.S., A.S., T.W., M.R., D.Y., R.S., V.R., N.F., C.B., J.A., A.C., D.D., and friends at the Southwestern Company.

Two groups deserve special recognition. Our families, immediate and extended, unselfishly gave time, patience, and understanding through many trying moments. Finally, we would like to acknowledge the thousands of courageous, dedicated men and women who are making their own heroic daily contributions to the fight against this disease.

J.I.S.
J.K.B.
Bethesda, Maryland
October 7, 1985

CONTENTS

I

THE AIDS EPIDEMIC: HOW YOU CAN PROTECT YOURSELF AND YOUR FAMILY

II

THE AIDS EPIDEMIC: PAST, PRESENT, AND FUTURE

I

THE AIDS EPIDEMIC: HOW YOU CAN PROTECT YOURSELF AND YOUR FAMILY

1

Who Should Be Concerned?

The AIDS epidemic has taken America by surprise. A generation previously unacquainted with fatal infectious diseases has been shocked by accounts of young people stricken by unexpected terminal illness. A nation accustomed to sexual license is fast becoming aware that intimate contact today carries with it the risk of life-threatening infection. Although the virus that causes AIDS came to America by 1977, the disease was not recognized or defined until June 1981. Five years later, in June 1986, AIDS will have claimed 10,000 American lives. Barring some currently unimaginable medical miracle, AIDS will claim 100,000 more lives in the five years that follow.

Physicians, often models of restraint in public pronouncements about disease, are speaking in apocalyptic terms. Dr. Alvin Friedman-Kien of the New York University Medical Center, one of the first physicians to diagnose AIDS, said, "If you were the devil, you couldn't conceive of a disease that would be more disruptive and disturbing than this one. It could prove to be the plague of the millennium." Dr. Ward Cates of the Centers for Disease Control, the federal agency responsible for tracking disease, said, "Anyone who has the least ability to look into the future can already see the potential for this disease being much worse than anything mankind has seen before."

The virus that causes AIDS is continually demonstrating its remarkable ability to conduct at the microscopic level a campaign of "germ" guerrilla warfare. It slips unnoticed into the bloodstreams of its victims, essentially causing no external signs or symptoms for a year or more. Despite this stealthy entry, the virus causes enormous medical and social complications for those it infects. Carriers are considered indefinitely infectious and, to completely protect their loved ones, should drastically alter their sex lives, reevaluate marriage plans, and eliminate the idea of conceiving children. Infected individuals are constantly threatened not only by the specter of developing AIDS, but also by the possibility that they may develop any of a number of cancers, blood malignancies, and neurological complications. In the near future they may be considered uninsurable by many companies and suffer serious employment consequences as well.

A great deal of the confusion surrounding this disease is related to the oft-repeated but mistaken notion that AIDS is somehow related to homosexuality. The large proportion of AIDS cases to date in gay men is due to an historic coincidence peculiar to the American pattern of AIDS virus spread. Unknown to anyone in America at the time, the virus was first introduced in this country into urban homosexual communities. Increased exposure in these communities to the virus solely accounts for the many AIDS cases diagnosed in homosexual and bisexual men. The virus has no intrinsic attraction for gays, and gays have no mysterious susceptibility to infection.

The pattern of African AIDS offers a compelling contrast. The virus was introduced in central Africa into heterosexual populations. The results are what one would expect from a sexually transmitted disease. *African AIDS correlates to upper-middle-class status, urban residence, heterosexual promiscuity, and contact with female prostitutes.* Further, the ratio of male to female AIDS cases in Africa is nearly 1 to 1. The virus clearly can be transmitted effectively from female to male, as well as from male to female or male to male. The conclusion is inescapable. AIDS is a potentially fatal venereal disease that threatens all sexually active people.

Dr. Robert Gallo of the National Cancer Institute, one of the world's foremost AIDS researchers, puts this into perspective:

There is nothing special about this virus by logic that should have said that this is a virus of homosexuals. We handled that question in that way in the beginning, but we never thought that there was anything that was special about homosexuals—*only that they were the group in the Western hemisphere that have the most contact with the virus, and keeping mostly to themselves it was confined in that population. Clearly the virus can go man-man, man-woman, woman-man* and I don't think there is a single bit of interest in the mode of sex. I think it was vastly overplayed and too much attention given it from day one. The virus will go man-woman, woman-man by more than one route. (Emphasis supplied.)

Individuals who continue to seize on the AIDS epidemic as a divine "punishment" for homosexuality are demonstrating their own ignorance. Heterosexuals who are tempted to be smug about their perceived exemption from this epidemic should consider the facts. One-fourth of all American AIDS victims to date have been heterosexuals. Today there are more than 250,000 infected American heterosexuals, 90% of whom are unaware of their own infection. Press coverage to the contrary notwithstanding, male-female and female-male transmission of the AIDS virus has been extensively documented. Although multiple sexual partners correlate most strongly to AIDS virus infection in heterosexuals, any partner of the past few years represents a possible source of infection.

Men who have contact with prostitutes and women who have intimate relations with bisexual men are emphatically at risk. Urban prostitutes particularly facilitate AIDS virus transmission. There may be 6,000 infected prostitutes in New York City alone and 40% of a group of Miami prostitutes were found to be infected. In some cities many of the sexually active bisexual men are infected as well.

In spite of the incontrovertible evidence relating to heterosexual spread of the AIDS virus, some individuals will undoubtedly cling to the cherished notion that AIDS is a homosexual disease. The continuing number of homosexual AIDS cases will supposedly "prove the point." It is important to remember that, due to the time lag (several years in most cases) between infection and the development of disease, *today's pattern of AIDS cases merely reflects the pattern of infection of two or more years ago.* AIDS virus infection has expanded in heterosexuals in America. Today there are at least as many infected heterosexual men and women as there were infected homosexual men in 1982. We can expect to see an explosion of heterosexual AIDS cases in the next few years.

A second "line of defense" often used to deflect personal concern about AIDS is the simplistic notion that science will soon develop a cure. Approximately half of the Americans alive today are under 35 years of age and have no recollection of the last fatal infectious disease—polio. While denial and disbelief are understandable reactions, the notion that medical science is on the verge of a breakthrough that will soon end this epidemic is dangerously delusional.

The truth is that those closest to the problem do not expect an effective treatment program or vaccine within the decade. Presently, an AIDS virus vaccine is inconceivable. Unlike the polio virus, the AIDS virus continually mutates. There have been 18 variants isolated, and were a vaccine developed, it would likely have effect on a limited number of variants for a limited amount of time. It took 11 years of concentrated research to develop a hepatitis B vaccine, and the AIDS virus is proving to be a much more complex medical challenge.

In spite of an unprecedented global research effort, AIDS has as yet proven impossible to treat. Although a number of experimental approaches have been tried, science has not been able to prolong the average life expectancy of the AIDS patient—18 months following diagnosis. Antiviral agents, often described as the greatest hope, have shown little or no relationship to clinical improvement in patients and often have toxic side effects that limit their potential usefulness as treatment. Immune boosters have also proven inadequate to the task of restoring a ravaged immune system. In addition, should a treatment program show promise, it will be subjected to the lengthy and tedious procedure of clinical trials, adding perhaps years to a timetable for making such therapy widely available.

Dr. Michael Gottlieb of the UCLA School of Medicine, widely known as Rock Hudson's American doctor, said, "The word cure *is not even in the vocabulary.*" (Emphasis supplied.) At a July Congressional hearing on funding for AIDS research, Dr. James Mason, Acting Assistant Secretary for Health, said that "although no stone was left unturned, a vaccine or treatment will not be available before 1990." Reporting on the April 1985 International Conference on AIDS in Atlanta, Marsha Goldsmith of the *Medical News* wrote, "Extremely guarded optimism about future victory over the disease by means of some yet undeveloped method of prevention and/or cure ran a poor second to the grimness of current battlefield dispatches."

In spite of the gloominess of the present situation, there are some hopeful signs. News of Rock Hudson's affliction and death have personalized AIDS for millions of Americans, fueling a growing awareness of the disease. Congress has approved an increase of more than 100% in federal funding for AIDS research, meaning that very little valuable basic science research for AIDS will be delayed due to lack of funding. Although the outlook on the medical horizon is not immediately promising, AIDS investigation is likely to have a number of long-term "spin-off" benefits in areas such as cancer and blood disease research.

The spread of AIDS virus infection is quite troubling. The AIDS virus is infecting Americans at the rate of one every 90 seconds. Some experts project that by the end of the decade 10 million, or perhaps double or triple that number, will be infected. On the other hand, even the most pessimistic do not project more than 2 to 3 million Americans are currently infected. *The vast majority of adults in this country, both homosexual and heterosexual, are not now infected with this virus.* Further, the means of transmission of the virus are well enough understood that *informed individuals can nearly eliminate their chances of infection by making responsible personal choices.*

Although the virus can be spread by a number of methods, sexual transmission will remain the threat to the greatest number of people. Uninfected individuals can take specific steps to protect themselves from infection. The number of partners should be greatly reduced, one should know one's partner before engaging in intimacies, and, unless both have had recent negative blood tests for the virus, some form of "safe sex" should be practiced. Although historically sexually transmitted diseases have been practically impossible to control, information from homosexual communities shows a massive drop in rates of all types of venereal disease. Hopefully, the rate of AIDS virus infection is slowing as well.

There are some welcome hints of good news for those currently infected. There is a growing body of evidence that following common-sense health practices (regular diet, sleep, moderate exercise, and avoiding infection) may reduce the chances of developing AIDS. Safe-sex practices apply to infected individuals as well, not only to protect uninfected partners, but also to prevent additional infections which may provoke an AIDS virus attack. Additionally, a public more fully informed about the harmlessness of casual contact will hopefully be less paranoid, more sympathetic and rational.

Every American is affected by the AIDS epidemic, which has become the greatest threat to public health in modern history. Those who believe themselves to be safe with an uninfected partner have friends, family, and loved ones at risk. AIDS threatens each of us in a personal way and our nation as well. If the spread of the virus were halted today—something that is clearly impossible—AIDS would still cost our nation $100 billion in direct outlays and lost earnings. With a projected doubling of new AIDS cases each year through the end of the decade, it is obvious that the day may come when AIDS threatens America's stability and prosperity.

History tells us that sexually transmitted diseases are impossible to control through government "crackdown." The spread of the virus must be stopped. *Education* and *personal sexual responsibility* are the only hope. In spite of intense media coverage of AIDS, the vast majority of Americans know very little about this disease. Television and news-magazine coverage aimed at educating typically lack the depth necessary to explain not only the facts about the AIDS epidemic but also the reasons behind them. Although unfolding developments prevent any written work to have the "last word" on AIDS, the information contained within should provide a comprehensive framework for understanding the complex range of issues created by this disease. To begin, it seems worthwhile to describe what science now knows about the incredible germ that causes AIDS.

2

What Causes AIDS and How Does It Work?

The microbial monster that arrived unannounced on the American shore in the late 1970s is invisible to the naked eye. The AIDS virus measures just 100–120 nanometers across.[1] It is so tiny that if 100,000 of them were laid end to end the result would barely be visible. It cannot even be detected with a normal (optical) microscope. It takes an electron microscope to photograph an AIDS virus in action. (See Figure 2–1.)

Despite its tiny size, the AIDS virus has proven itself to be one of the most deadly germs to ever infect humans. It is a tiny killing machine of almost unbelievable durability and potency. It has the ability to disguise itself within a cell. Once inside a body, it cannot be killed by any known medical means. It can launch a preemptive strike on the immune system, which is the body's way of defending itself from *all kinds* of germs. It can enlist a wide variety of other germs and give them a clear field in which to attack and kill.

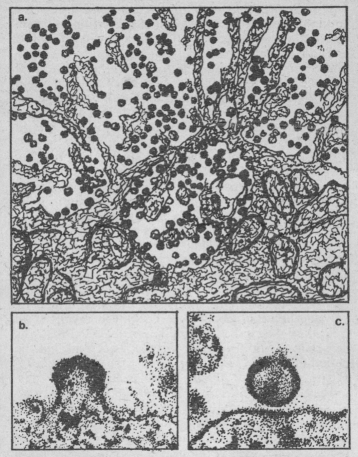

Figure 2-1. (a.) T-helper cell is surrounded by newly formed AIDS viruses.(black dots).(b.) New viruses form by budding from cell surface.(c.) Newly formed AIDS viruses, manufactured in cell, break free, searching for a new T-helper cell.

There is an evolutionary process that takes place in the germ world much like the process of adaptation and natural selection first described by Charles Darwin in the plant and animal world. Over time, the more successful adaptations survive and thrive. The AIDS virus is a miniature example of an evolutionary "success story." It has the ability to slightly alter its structure over time. It has adapted so successfully to its microbial environment that it now represents the most refined example of a family of killer germs known as retroviruses.

Other members of the retrovirus family are germs that cause leukemia in a number of animals (including leukemia in cats). The first *human* retrovirus was identified by Dr. Robert Gallo of the National Cancer Institute in 1978.[2] This virus, known technically as human T-cell leukemia virus, or HTLV-I, was the first germ ever clearly identified as the primary cause of human cancer.[3]

Retroviruses have proven to be remarkable for their virulence (deadly nature) and for their endurance. Retroviruses are the cause of a number of lethal blood malignancies. HTLV-I causes leukemia in humans and is particularly prevalent in certain populations of southern Japan, central Africa, the West Indies, and southeastern United States. Its persistence is amply demonstrated by the fact that the period between HTLV-I infection and the onset of leukemia is typically 15 to 20 years but can be as long as 40 years.

The AIDS virus, known as HTLV-III (human T-cell lymphotropic virus, type III),[4] is proving to be the most dangerous member of the retrovirus family. The AIDS virus can arrive in the bloodstream by a number of different routes, and becomes so prevalent within an infected individual that it permeates the blood, semen, saliva, urine, and tears.[5-11] Any exchange of these fluids between an infected and an uninfected individual is risky, though the risk varies with the amount and type of fluid exchanged. (See question 9.)

Upon entering a new bloodstream, the AIDS virus looks for a place to "set up shop." It targets many cells, but most significantly the T-helper cell, a type of white blood cell.[12] This particular cell is considered to be the worst possible cell for the virus to attack.

In the bloodstreams of healthy individuals, there are white blood cells to seek out, locate, and destroy hostile invading germs. There exist various types of white blood cells, each of which has a specific and necessary role to play in a functioning immune system. One type, dendritic macrophages (radar) perform reconnaissance and early warning functions. (See Figure 2–2.) These reconnaissance cells are located in the liver and spleen and aggressively search for foreign germs. When they locate an invading microbe, they send out a chemical signal that acts as the first sign of trouble.

This signal is understood by the T-helper cells, the "field generals" making up the "field command structure" of the body's defense system. They sound a general alarm, launching a full-scale alert, mobilization, and attack. The T-helper cells send out the signal to the various units of the body's defense. Upon receiving this signal, the body's immune system begins to deploy T-killer cells (commandos) to locate the invaders and cause B-attack cells to manufacture and fire weapons (tanks, machine guns, planes, missiles) necessary to destroy the foreign germs. Phagocytic cells (infantry) are sent to devour and mop up the enemy.

Without the T-helper cells sounding the general alarm, the resources to repel an invasion of foreign germs cannot be mobilized. Thus the immune system is dysfunctional. In the absence of a functioning immune system, germs that would normally be identified, tracked down, and rendered harmless are allowed to continue along their course unopposed, thus becoming life threatening. This is precisely what happens in end-stage AIDS patients.

This does not happen immediately, or even soon after an AIDS virus first invades a victim's bloodstream. As soon as an AIDS virus enters a new bloodstream, it locates a specific T-helper cell. The virus has a method of incorporating itself within the genetic structure of a T-helper cell. (See

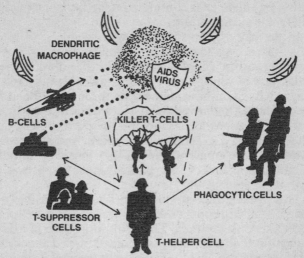

Figure 2-2. The body's immune system mobilizes against an
AIDS virus attack.

Figure 2–3.) This process does not kill a T-helper cell, but
renders it unable to perform its function as "field general"
of the immune system. A T-helper cell that has been invaded by an AIDS virus cannot sound the alarm to the rest
of the body's immune system.[13-16] One useful way of pictur-
ing this is that the "field general" has been "taken hostage"
but not killed.

The invasion and "hostage-taking" of one T-helper cell
does not, by itself, render a person's immune system unable
to function. There are millions of other functioning T-
helper cells which can do the job. The sinister effect this
has, though, is that it makes the presence of the AIDS virus
covert and unrecognizable. Most people who have been
infected with the AIDS virus are not aware of it for at least

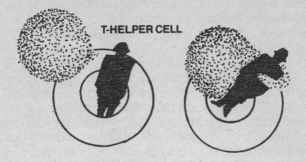

Figure 2-3. AIDS virus captures T-helper cell.

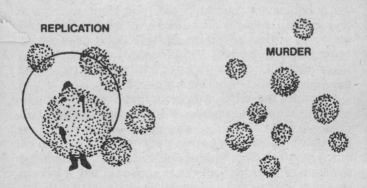

Figure 2-4.(a.) The AIDS virus turns the T-helper cell into a replicative factory.(b.) The AIDS virus kills the T-helper cell, after having produced millions of replicas of itself.

one year. During this period of "dormancy," the AIDS virus has not attacked enough T-helper cells to cause noticeable damage to the immune system.

While some T-helper cells are immobilized by AIDS virus attack, the remaining healthy "field generals" signal "attack-type" B-cells to release proteins called *antibodies* —biological "bullets" which are fired at the invading germs. For example, when measles viruses invade a bloodstream for the first time the dendritic macrophages sense them and sound the preliminary alarm, which is picked up by the T-helper cells. Measles antibodies are produced that destroy the measles germs. A "battle" takes place over a period of time as antibodies are fired. While the "battle" is taking place, the infected individual goes through the external signs and symptoms of measles. Over a period of a few weeks, the measles germs are eventually killed, the external signs and symptoms go away, and the body's immune system returns to normal.

Antibodies are specific to the type of germ they are trying to k . Measles antibodies are different, for example, from tibodies to the Epstein-Barr virus (which causes mononucleosis). That the body can produce so many different, specific types of antibodies is one of the miracles of a functioning immune system.

Incredibly, the AIDS virus seems impervious to the antibodies that the body produces to combat it. The AIDS virus seems to be a killer with armor-plated protection against which the immune system's "bullets" have no effect. The AIDS virus has sheltered itself within the genetic structure of a T-helper cell and cannot be killed. It lurks in that form apparently indefinitely. There it remains, threatening to explode into an active phase of replication and to attack more T-helper cells.

The AIDS virus in a period of dormancy is holding one of the immune system's generals hostage with one hand on the throat and another with a gun held to the head. The general is not dead but is unable to perform traditional organizational functions. This period of dormancy ends when the "gun is fired." (See Figure 2–4.) When the AIDS virus explodes out of dormancy, it turns the host cell into a replicative factory. The AIDS virus uses the material of the invaded T-helper cell to manufacture millions of copies of itself during the six hours prior to the host cell's death. These newly created AIDS viruses can then swim freely in the bloodstream to locate other healthy T-helper cells to invade and destroy.

The AIDS virus apparently has the "patience" to "hide out" for a seemingly indefinite period of time before starting to replicate. While the AIDS virus is in a period of dormancy it does little damage to the immune system. Thus the host is unaware that he or she has been infected. This is the state of the symptomless carrier.

Replication can be triggered by any number of medical events such as pregnancy, surgery, or concurrent stressful illnesses. These triggering influences are referred to as "cofactors." Notwithstanding the effect of cofactors, the virus itself is powerful enough to destroy a host. Thus the host lives under the double lifetime threat of replicative attack spurred by *agents provocateurs* (cofactors), or the spontaneous outbreak of the latent but ever-seething virus.

As the virus kills and captures the command structure of a body's immune system, there are fewer and fewer T-helper cells floating around. As a person progresses through the stages of immune attack, an analysis of his or her blood will indicate fewer and fewer T-helper cells. The blood becomes "thinner and thinner." The AIDS virus has thus "executed its mission" and killed most of the "field generals."

The AIDS virus can do more than destroy a functioning immune system. It also recruits a variety of deadly support troops in the form of other germs. A dysfunctional immune system will not, by itself, kill a person. It renders them defenseless against attack by other germs. The AIDS virus achieves unilateral disarmament of the body's weapons against disease. An individual thus disarmed an open invitation to microbial assault.

This process feeds on itself. The weaker a person's immune system becomes, the more inviting a target it becomes for other infections. The more it is attacked by new germs, the weaker it becomes. In the terminal stages AIDS, patients are victimized by unrelenting, multiple infections. People who die of AIDS actually die of the complications of unopposed infection caused by this assemblage of germs.

Pneumocystis carinii is a protozoan (parasite) that attacks the lungs of most AIDS patients,[17-18] causing pneumonia. *Pneumocystis* infection results in persistent fever, cough, and shortness of breath. Victimized patients usually survive the first attack of *Pneumocystis carinii*, but it frequently reappears and is often part of the cause death.

Another "ally" often recruited by the AIDS virus *Toxoplasmosis gondii*.[18] Toxoplasmosis is a protozoan that attacks the eyes, heart, and central nervous system. It evidenced by fever and signs of neurological deterioration such as loss of memory and loss of orientation. *Cryptosporidium* is yet another protozoan that can cause unrelenting watery diarrhea in patients with AIDS or AIDS-related complex.[18]

Candidiasis is a fungus that often painfully attacks the throat area, causing cheesy white deposits.[18] *Cryptococcus neoformans* is a devastating fungus that attacks the lungs, central nervous system, lymph nodes, intestinal tract, and bone marrow. It can also infect the cerebrospinal fluid individuals.[18]

A number of bacteria also attack people with immune systems damaged by the AIDS virus. Two of these are *Mycobacterium avium-intracellulare* and *Mycobacterium tuberculosis*. These germs cause different types of tuberculosis.[18]

Many viruses serve as the "support troops" recruited the deadly AIDS virus. One of these is cytomegalovirus common but usually harmless germ, which, with the help of the AIDS virus, attacks the lungs, central nervous system, liver, intestines, and urinary tract and is the most common cause of death of AIDS patients.[18] Cytomegalovirus belongs to the herpes family of viruses. It can cause blindness, pneumonia, hepatitis, colitis, and encephalitis. Herpes simplex and herpes zoster are other viruses that attack immune-deficient patients.[18]

Another virus of the herpes family is the Epstein-Barr virus, which can cause cancer of the nose and throat, lymphoma, and mononucleosis.[19] Indeed, some of the most common allies recruited by the AIDS virus are cancers.[20] Kaposi's sarcoma, a previously rare form of skin cancer causing purplish or reddish lesions over the legs of elderly men of Italian or Eastern European Jewish ancestry, is common in AIDS patients.

Kaposi's sarcoma in AIDS patients is more aggressive than the classic form described by the Hungarian dermatologist Moriz Kaposi?[21] AIDS-related Kaposi's sarcoma is characterized by the sudden and often widespread occurrence of cancerous lesions involving the skin, lining of the mouth, lymph glands, and many internal organs, such as the liver, spleen, lung, and gastrointestinal tract.

Hodgkin's disease and non-Hodgkin's lymphoma (cancer of the glands) also attack individuals who have immune systems weakened by the AIDS virus.[22-24] It is worth noting that the AIDS virus and its microbial allies are so powerful that the cancers they cause are rarely the cause of death of AIDS patients. AIDS patients usually die of opportunistic infections, which in concert with the AIDS virus can kill more rapidly than cancer.

Unfortunately, none of this was known when the AIDS virus first made its way to American shores. It had a free ride of several years. By the time physicians were even aware of its extraordinary work, the AIDS virus had established a beachhead in America. It had infected thousands of people, beginning in male homosexuals and working its way silently to other groups. (Simultaneously, it was spreading prolifically in Africa through heterosexual contact.) American physicians thus were surprised in the spring of 1981 when previously rare diseases typical of people with impaired immune systems began appearing in a number of previously healthy young men.

CHAPTER 2 REFERENCES

1. Barre-Sinoussi F, Chermann JC, Rey F, et al. Isolation of T-lymphotropic retrovirus from a patient at risk from acquired immune deficiency syndrome (AIDS). Science 220:868, 1983.

2. Poiesz BJ, Ruscetti FW, Gazdar AF, et al. Detection and isolation of type C retrovirus particles from fresh and cultured lymphocytes of a patient with cutaneous T-cell lymphoma. Proc Natl Acad Sci USA 77:7415, 1980.

3. Broder S, Bunn PA, Jaffee ES, et al. T-cell lymphoproliferative syndrome associated with human T-cell leukemia/lymphoma virus. Ann Intern Med 100:543, 1984.

4. Broder S, Gallo RC. A pathogenic retrovirus (HTLV-III) linked to AIDS. N Engl J Med 311:1292, 1984.

5. Curran JW, Lawrence DN, Jaffee H, et al. Acquired immunodeficiency syndrome associated with transfusions. N Engl J Med 310:69, 1984.

6. Jaffe HW, Francis DP, McLane MF, et al. Transfusion-associated AIDS: Serologic evidence of human T-cell leukemia virus infection of donors. Science 223:1309, 1984.

7. Gallo RC, Salahuddin SZ, Popovic M, et al. Frequent detection and isolation of cytopathic retroviruses (HTLV-III) from patients with AIDS and at risk for AIDS. Science 224:500, 1984.

8. Zagury D, Bernard J, Leibowitch J, et al. HTLV-III in cells cultured from semen of two patients with AIDS. Science 226:449, 1984.

9. Ho DD, Schooley RT, Rota TR, et al. HTLV-III in the semen and blood of a healthy homosexual man. Science 226:451, 1984.

10. Groopman JE, Salahuddin SZ, Sarngadharan MG, et al. HTLV- III in saliva of people with AIDS-related complex and healthy homosexual men at risk for AIDS. Science 226:447, 1984.

11. Fujikawa LS, Palestine AG, Nussenblatt RB, et al. Isolation of human T-lymphotropic virus type III from the tears of a patient with the acquired immunodeficiency syndrome. Lancet 2:529, 1985.

12. Fauci AS, Macher AM, Longo DL, et al. Acquired immunodeficiency syndrome: Epidemiologic, clinical, immunologic, and therapeutic considerations. Ann Intern Med 100:92, 1984.

13. Gallo RC, Shaw GM, Markham PD. The etiology of AIDS. In *AIDS: Etiology, Diagnosis, Treatment, and Prevention*. DeVita VT, Hellman S, Rosenberg SA (eds). J.B. Lippincott Company, New York, p. 31-54, 1985.

14. Lane HC, Depper JM, Greene WC, et al. Qualitative analysis of immune function in patients with the acquired immunodeficiency syndrome: evidence for a selective defect in soluble antigen recognition. N Engl J Med 313:79, 1985.

15. Kalish RS, Schlossman SF. The T4 lymphocyte in AIDS. N Engl J Med 313:112, 1985.

16. Fauci AS. Immunologic abnormalities in the acquired immunodeficiency syndrome. Clin Res 32 no 5:491, 1984.

17. Goedert JJ, Blattner WA. The epidemiology of AIDS and related conditions. In *AIDS: Etiology, Diagnosis, Treatment, and Prevention*. DeVita VT, Hellman S, Rosenberg SA (eds). J.B. Lippincott Company, New York, p. 1-30, 1985.

18. Masur H, Kovacs, JA, Ognibene F, et al. Infectious complications of AIDS. In *AIDS: Etiology, Diagnosis, Treatment, and Prevention*. DeVita VT, Hellman S, Rosenberg SA (eds). J.B. Lippincott Company, New York, p. 161-184, 1985.

19. Lipscomb H, Tatsurmi E, Harada S, et al. Epstein-Barr virus and chronic lymphadenomegaly in male homosexual with acquired immunodeficiency syndrome. AIDS Res 1:59, 1983.

20. Safi B, Koziner B. Malignant neoplasms in AIDS. In *AIDS: Etiology, Diagnosis, Treatment, and Prevention*. DeVita VT, Hellman S, Rosenberg SA (eds). J.B. Lippincott Company, New York, p. 213-222, 1985.

21. Kaposi M. Classics in oncology: Idiopathic multiple pigmented sarcoma of the skin. (Translated and reprinted.) CA 32:342, 1982.
22. Ziegler JL, Beckstead JA, Volberding PA, et al. Non-Hodgkin's lymphoma in 90 homosexual men. N Engl J Med 311:565, 1984.
23. Levine AM, Meyer RR, Begandy MK, et al. Development of B-cell lymphoma in homosexual men. Ann Intern Med 100:7, 1984.
24. Dancis A, Odajnyk C, Kriegel RL, et al. Association of Hodgkin's and non-Hodgkin's lymphomas with the acquired immunodeficiency syndrome (AIDS). Proc Am Soc Clin Oncol 3:61a (c 236), 1984.

3

The 100 Most Important Questions About AIDS

"HOW DO PEOPLE BECOME INFECTED?"

1. **Q.** Where, when and how did the first human become infected with the AIDS virus?

   A. It is difficult to be precise about this. Best estimates show pockets of AIDS virus infection in eastern Africa in the early 1970s. It is believed that the disease came to man from green monkeys *(Cercopithecus aethiops)*. Unlike man, green monkeys can carry the virus without it destroying their immune system.

   Green monkeys have apparently evolved a means to control the virus, according to Dr. Max Essex of the Harvard School of Public Health. It is possible that by studying this mechanism it could be of help in the battle against AIDS, most particularly in the development of a vaccine. However, it is not expected that this will lead to a tangible treatment for AIDS or a vaccine for the AIDS virus anytime soon.

2. **Q. When and how did AIDS come to America?**

A. Acquired immune deficiency syndrome was first defined by the Centers for Disease Control in June 1981. After more was known about AIDS, past medical records were examined. Fifty-seven cases were reclassified and defined as AIDS previous to 1981. There were 4 cases of AIDS in 1978, 9 cases in 1979, and 44 cases in 1980.

There is a time lag of one year or more between infection with the AIDS virus and the development of signs or symptoms of AIDS. It is believed that the virus first infected Americans in either 1976 or 1977.

It is believed that the first Americans infected were tourists vacationing in the Caribbean. The virus came to the Caribbean from Africa in the middle 1970s. It is believed that the virus first entered America in urban areas of New York City, Miami, Los Angeles, and San Francisco. (See Figure 3–1.)

3. **Q. Is the AIDS virus contagious?**

A. Yes. The virus has been transmitted between male homosexuals, between heterosexuals, between intravenous drug users sharing contaminated needles, from blood transfusions, from contaminated blood products, as well as from mother to infant.

4. **Q. How many people are infected with the AIDS virus?**

A. Until large numbers of Americans from a wide sampling of populations take the blood test, it will be hard to be certain. Current estimates run from a low of 500,000 to 3 million or more. CDC estimates published in August 1985 are illustrated in Figure 3–2.

AIDS is a sexually transmitted disease that has

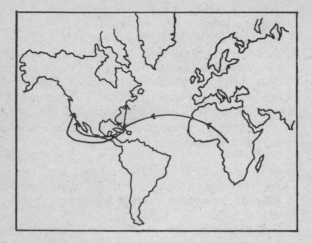

Figure 3-1. Spread of AIDS virus to the United States.

the ability to infect large numbers of people in
short periods of time. The AIDS virus achieved a
"portal of entry" into the San Francisco male homosexual community in the 1970s—probably 1976
or 1977. The virus was detected in only 1% of the
men attending a clinic for sexually transmitted
diseases in San Francisco in 1978. By 1980 the figure had grown to 25%, and by 1984 it was 65%.

The AIDS virus has no doubt achieved "portals
of entry" into a number of promiscuous heterosexual circles. A group of 25 prostitutes was sampled
in Miami and 10 (40%) were infected.[1] There are
likely 6,000 or more infected prostitutes in New
York City alone. Unless a major change is made in
heterosexual lifestyles, the AIDS virus may become as prevalent as herpes. Herpes was barely
even heard of in the 1950s. Its spread was widely

TOTAL NUMBER INFECTED

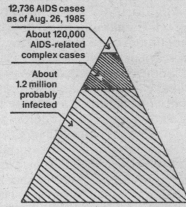

12,736 AIDS cases
as of Aug. 26, 1985

About 120,000
AIDS-related
complex cases

About
1.2 million
probably
infected

Figure 3-2. Estimates represent upper ranges of Centers for Disease Control projections.

publicized in the 1970s. By this year, 1985, it is estimated that 20 million Americans will have gotten genital herpes.

5. Q. **It is said that there are a million or more Americans who carry the AIDS virus, most of whom are symptomless. How infectious are these people?**

A. This is not known. The AIDS virus can be cultured from the blood, semen, tears, saliva, and urine of a large majority of these infected individuals. For this reason, individuals who are known to have the virus should refrain from sexual activity, including French kissing. (See also question 9.)

The AIDS virus is a member of a family of germs known as retroviruses. Once a retrovirus infects an individual, it becomes a permanent part of the host's genes. It may lie dormant with a low level of infectivity. If this proves to be the case, it means that infected people could have periods where they are less infectious. This is a pattern that has been observed in herpes.

The AIDS virus will suddenly burst forth in a phase of active replication after lying dormant for a period of time. The factors that "trigger" this active phase are unknown but may include such co-factors as other viral infections or significant medical crises. It is likely that an individual will be more infectious in this active phase than during the period of dormancy. The question of whether or not symptomless carriers have times of greater or less infectivity is one of the important questions about the AIDS virus. Until this is answered, people who have the AIDS virus should consider themselves indefinitely infectious. Harvard's Dr. William Haseltine put it this way: "Once infected, a person is infected for the rest of his life. Once infected, a person is *infectious*. It's not safe to assume otherwise."

6. Q. **Can you tell by inspecting a potential partner if that person carries the AIDS virus?**

   A. No. Unlike herpes, which may cause symptoms or signs such as pain or blisters, the symptomless carriers (which currently account for the vast majority of individuals who have been infected by the AIDS virus) *show no evidence of infection*. Tragically, most carriers are unaware that they have been infected by the AIDS virus and that they may be contagious. The only way for you to find out if you or a partner has been infected is to get your blood tested.

7. Q. **Can the symptomless carrier transmit full-blown AIDS?**

   A. Yes. One of the most heartbreaking aspects of the entire AIDS epidemic is that the symptomless carriers, who are unaware of the fact that they carry the AIDS virus, may unintentionally harm or kill the ones they love the most.

This depressing possibility is illustrated in the case of Patrick and Lauren Burk and their son of Cresson, Pennsylvania. The Burks were married in 1983 and were overjoyed at the birth of their son, Dwight, in April 1984. Medical complications arose that summer, and it was determined that all three were infected with the AIDS virus. Patrick received the AIDS virus from Factor VIII, a blood product he used because he is a hemophiliac.

All three have developed AIDS or AIDS-related complex, which means that the medical outlook for the next five years is gloomy at best. None may survive that period of time.

8. **Q. Will a vaccine be developed that will protect me against the AIDS virus?**

A. Possibly. The search for a vaccine is one of the hopeful areas in which to concentrate research efforts. Work on a vaccine is being conducted at the National Cancer Institute's Frederick Cancer Research Facility in Frederick, Maryland. However, the obstacles to a vaccine are, to say the least, formidable. It would be a severe mistake to base any future plans on the idea that a vaccination will appear anytime soon.

There are at least 18 different variants of the AIDS virus. It is also apparent that the virus mutates over time. If a vaccine were developed, it might be effective for a limited number of variants or for a limited amount of time.

One of the leading investigators at the respected Centers for Disease Control, Dr. James Curran, says this about the effort to develop a vaccine:

There is no evidence of a natural immunity (to the AIDS virus), and parts of the virus' genetic structure appear to be variable. That is bothersome to many scientists because that means a

vaccine might not be effective against all strains
of the virus.

Development of a vaccination will require
major advances in biomedical techniques. Even if
the necessary tools were achieved tomorrow, the
availability of a vaccine for public use would still
be years away. A vaccination would certainly be a
tremendous breakthrough. However, by the time a
vaccine might be developed, it is likely that several
million Americans will have been infected with
the AIDS virus. Dr. Curran has predicted that by
the time an effective vaccine is developed, it will
probably be necessary to vaccinate all Americans
before they become sexually active. For the foreseeable future, personal sexual responsibility is the
only effective way to counter the spread of the
AIDS virus.

9. Q. **What issues appear to be the most important in
   successful transmission of the AIDS virus?**
   A. There are three factors generally discussed as in-
   fluencing the possibility that a particular exposure will lead to AIDS virus infection: mode of
   transmission, dose of contagion, and condition of
   host at the time of exposure. The mode of transmission relates to the type of body fluid that is
   exchanged and the point at which it enters the host.
   Types of infected body fluid include the blood,
   semen, saliva, tears, and urine. Points of entry
   include the rectum, mouth, vagina, other mucosal
   membranes, blood vessels, and skin abrasions.
   Dose of contagion. In many infectious diseases
   there is a threshold value of contagion that must be
   present for infection to take place. This is referred
   to as "critical mass." The dose of AIDS virus contagion is related to the concentration of virus in the
   body fluid and the amount of fluid exchanged.
   Concentration of the virus varies within an indi-

vidual in the various fluids—semen, blood, saliva, tears, and urine. Volume relates to the amount of fluid exchanged—a large amount of semen presents a greater risk, for example.

Condition of host at time of exposure. Is he or she healthy? It appears that an activated immune system due to illness at the time of exposure may increase the chances for transmission. What is the state of his or her immune system? A weak or strained immune system (perhaps caused by an unrelated medical condition, trauma, or aging) increases susceptibility to infection. (See pp. 102–103.)

10. Q. Is kissing safe?

A. No. Current United States Food and Drug Administration and World Health Organization guidelines to individuals who have had a positive blood test showing antibodies to the AIDS virus specifically recommend that infected individuals refrain from intimate, or "French" kissing.

It is significant to appreciate that this was not always the case. Recommendations in 1983 did not mention intimate kissing as a possible form of virus transmission. However, since then the AIDS virus has been cultured out of the saliva of infected individuals. It is therefore reasonable to presume that infection could occur from the exchange of saliva which takes place in this form of sexual expression. This presumption is strengthened by a recent report of a case in which a woman developed AIDS virus infection. Her only identifiable risk was kissing her AIDS-patient husband.

It has been suggested that intimate kissing may be a lower risk activity than sexual practices in which other body fluids are exchanged. Given the available evidence, intimate kissing should be considered a risky activity by infected and uninfected individuals alike.(See pp. 102–103.)

11. Q. Other than through sexual contact, how can I catch the AIDS virus?

A. The other major mode of transmission is through contaminated blood or blood products. For this reason, it is possible to become infected with the AIDS virus by sharing an intravenous needle, a tattoo needle, an acupuncture needle, a razor, an electrolysis needle, or a needle to pierce your ears. It is believed that needles can probably be rendered safe for reuse by steam sterilization. However, it is better to avoid the possibility by using disposable needles.

The virus has also been transmitted from mother to unborn child (through the placenta) and to infant (through infected mother's milk).

12. Q. Am I safe, for example, in a restaurant, a bar, a Jacuzzi, a hot tub, or a public toilet?

A. Except for an unusual circumstance, a restaurant can be made safe through the disciplined application of basic sanitation procedures. If the plates, glasses, and utensils are washed with soap and water, this should kill any AIDS virus. An "unusual circumstance" might be an infected waiter or waitress spitting, sneezing, or bleeding on a plate of prepared food.

A bar is considered to be generally safe. It is unlikely that you could be infected with the virus from sipping the drink of an infected individual, though clearly this is not a good idea. Also, it is unclear if the "quick cleaning" procedure used in some bars is a completely effective way of killing the virus.

It is doubtful you could catch the AIDS virus in a hot tub or Jacuzzi. Because the water is chemically treated, it is unlikely to contain transmissible virus. However, in studies of herpes the plastic surfaces have been found to have live germs for short periods of time. It is unclear whether the AIDS virus can live in this setting.

The danger posed by a public toilet seat is quite small. It is possible for a seat to be contaminated by the saliva, semen, blood, or urine of an infected individual. The survival period of the AIDS virus outside the body is unknown. Even if the virus survives long enough for the next occupant of the toilet seat to sit down, it would need a portal such as a bleeding hemorrhoid, pimple, or rectal irritation to the bloodstream. Although scientific precaution dictates the delineation of these possible methods of transmission, the authors believe the actual threat to the individual is comparable to being hit with a bolt of lightning.

13. Q. **Can I catch the AIDS virus from sharing a drink, a cigarette, or a marijuana joint with an infected individual?**

A. Probably not. Although the AIDS virus has been cultivated from the saliva of infected individuals, it is unlikely that it could be transmitted from the sharing of a drink, cigarette, or marijuana joint.

The heat of a cigarette or joint might be enough to kill the virus. However, if a substantial amount of saliva was left on the paper this might not be true. The alcohol contained in a drink might also be able to kill the virus.

Additionally, if infected saliva was swallowed, it would likely need a portal to the bloodstream. The AIDS virus seems to act like the hepatitis virus, which is believed to be killed by the acidic secretions of a normal digestive system. However, a cut lip, canker sore, fever blister, or injured gum could provide such a portal.

Although the probability of being infected by any of these routes is low, eliminating the possibility as a precautionary measure is a good idea.

14. Q. **Is my child safe from the AIDS virus at school?**

A. Most likely. The AIDS virus has been observed in adults and infants as a result of parental infection. It is very rare in school-age children, even those in areas where the virus is known to be prevalent. There is little evidence to support the idea that the virus can be transmitted through casual contact in a school setting.

We could look at the "dark side" and note that in certain schools there is a severe drug problem. It is conceivable that a child could receive the AIDS virus through having shared a needle with an infected individual. There has also been a dramatic increase in sexual activity and sexual abuse in our nation's schools. These are situations in which there may be risk of AIDS virus infection. But there are no recorded examples of children having received the AIDS virus from casual contact experienced in normal school activities.

15. Q. **Is my son or daughter safe at college?**
    A. Possibly. If your son or daughter refrains from sex and needle sharing, he or she is safe at college.

Although it has been said many times, it bears repeating that casual contact (sharing a living space, classroom, cafeteria table) does not create risk for contracting the AIDS virus. However, there are some characteristics of college and university towns that are favorable to the spread of AIDS virus infection.

Many university towns have a high rate of sexual activity, and students come from all over the world. Students who come from areas of high prevalence of AIDS virus infection may be symptomless carriers with the potential to infect others, starting a wave of contagion. Colleges and universities surrounding large cities are also susceptible to initial infections from outside influences, namely infected urban dwellers. The AIDS virus has shown remarkable ability to spread throughout promiscuous communities. (Infection among sexually active San Francisco men jumped from 1% in 1978 to 65% in 1984.)

Some colleges also have a problem with intravenous drug use. Students who share intravenous needles are at risk for contracting the virus. College students should be advised to refrain from practices involving sharing of needles, reduce their number of sexual partners, and practice "safe sex."

16. Q. Are many female prostitutes infected, and are they a risk to their customers?

A. Yes. Contact with prostitutes is a risk factor for AIDS virus infection all over the world. A study of Rwanda (Africa) prostitutes showed that 88% were infected. Rwandan men who frequent prostitutes are four times more likely to be infected than other sexually active Rwandan men.

In Miami, 40% of a group of prostitutes was found to be infected.[1] Many cities have a large number of prostitutes infected by contaminated needles. It has been estimated that there are 100,000 to 200,000 intravenous drug abusers in the metropolitan New York City area.[2] Twenty percent of intravenous drug users are women, of which one-third admit to prostitution.[3] There may be 6,000 or more infected female prostitutes in New York due to the use of contaminated needles.

17. Q. Can mosquitoes spread the virus?

A. Unlikely. This question is being investigated in the United States in the small community of Belle Glade, Florida. In that agricultural town in south central Florida, there were 37 cases of AIDS reported through March 1985 in a community of 17,000. There may be 1,000 or more infected residents.

Belle Glade is unlike the urban settings in the United States in which the AIDS virus has proliferated. It is an impoverished agricultural area in which overcrowding, malnutrition, venereal disease, and tuberculosis are common; quite similar to the settings in Africa in which the AIDS virus is prevalent.

Significantly more than half of the first 37 cases reported did not fit into any of the high-risk categories. In these cases the source and agent of transmission in Belle Glade is undefined. It has been suggested that mosquitoes may provide a clue. It is hypothetically possible but unlikely that if a mosquito bites an infected individual and then an uninfected individual, the virus could be transmitted. However, at present, this mode of transmission has not been established.

18. Q. Can I catch the AIDS virus by shaking hands with an infected person?

A. Probably not. Although colds have been transmitted at times by shaking hands, this is not a way to catch the AIDS virus. There is very little evidence to suggest you can transmit or receive the AIDS virus from "casual contact." For example, there are no recorded examples in this country of someone who has AIDS in a household transmitting it to someone else in the household from hugging, touching, or sitting nearby. The household transmissions have been through either sexual contact, sharing of needles (as with intravenous drug users), or from mother to infant or unborn child.

19. Q. Can I catch the AIDS virus from infected sweat or tears?

A. Possibly, though not likely.

Dr. Zaki Salahuddin has isolated AIDS virus from the tears of infected individuals. There is a high concentration of white blood cells in tears, and so this discovery is not particularly surprising. The chances of contracting the AIDS virus from contact with infected tears is quite low. It would likely require infected tears to come into contact with a portal to the bloodstream, such as an open cut or abrasion.

The AIDS virus has not been cultured from the perspiration of infected individuals. There are few white blood cells in sweat, and the saline concentration would likely retard any AIDS virus which might be present.

20. Q. Can I catch the AIDS virus from my barber or hairdresser?

A. Probably not. Presuming you refrain from sexual contact or the sharing of infected needles, you are safe. The rare exception might be an infected barber or hairdresser whose cut finger bleeds into a portion of scalp which is raw from irritation. This could be safely said to be an extremely unusual situation, presenting little, if any, danger.

21. Q. Can I catch the AIDS virus by wearing the clothes of an infected person?

A. No. There is no evidence that the AIDS virus can be transmitted through wearing the clothes of an infected person. Naturally, it would be a good idea to wash the clothes before wearing them.

22. Q. Can I catch the AIDS virus from food in a grocery store or from a contaminated water supply?

A. No. The AIDS virus can be transmitted sexually, through the blood, or through the sharing of infected needles. AIDS virus contagion does not survive outside an infected individual in sufficient quantity to be transmitted through food in a grocery store. The precautions that are currently prescribed by local health departments are quite sufficient to see to it that the AIDS virus cannot be transmitted through the water supply.

23. Q. Can a newborn infant become infected with the AIDS virus by sharing nursery space with an infant infected with the AIDS virus?

A. No. The virus cannot be transmitted simply by the sharing of nursery space with an infected infant.

24. Q. How do infants become infected?

   A. Infants can become infected with the AIDS virus
   through the placenta, or through drinking an infected mother's milk. Examples of "pediatric
   AIDS" are becoming more prevalent. In New York
   City alone, an average of two infants per day are
   born to mothers who have the AIDS virus. Couples
   planning to have children should consider having
   their blood tested for the AIDS virus.

**25. Q. What was the source of concern that former Geor-
   gia Governor Lester Maddox had been infected?**

   A. Former Governor Maddox had been treated for
   cancer at a clinic in the Bahamas that was subsequently closed due to AIDS virus infection in
   serum samples. The Immunology Researching
   Center Ltd. in Freeport was closed by the Baha-
   mian government July 17, 1985, when officials
   found AIDS virus antibodies in 18 vials of blood.

   Former Governor Maddox had received more
   than 60 serum injections from the clinic. When the
   discovery of AIDS virus contamination was announced, it was feared that he may have been infected.

**26. Q. Can a woman be infected by artificial insemina-
   tion?**

   A. Yes. Four cases of AIDS virus infection related to
   artificial insemination have been reported in Australia. Three of the four women are symptomless,
   and one has swollen glands, a symptom of ARC.
   All four were infected from sperm obtained from
   the same donor. It should be noted that these
   women were infected in 1982, before the AIDS
   virus had been identified or a test developed to
   detect its presence.

   The Australian sperm banks were closed by the
   government in November 1984 due to this problem
   and reopened in April 1985 with strict AIDS virus
   screening procedures put in place. Letters were

sent to all women who had been inseminated at the facility that had the infected semen. Eighty percent responded and tests showed that none of them were infected. The Food and Drug Administration's guidelines in effect in America should practically eliminate the possibility of a similar incident occurring in this country.

27. Q. Am I safe if I receive an organ transplant?

A. Probably. Food and Drug Administration guidelines recommend that all donated organs be checked for the AIDS virus by having the donor's blood tissue analyzed. This testing will practically eliminate the possibility of being infected via a donated organ. There is only one recorded example of an infected organ (a kidney) in America causing AIDS virus infection.

28. Q. Can I catch the AIDS virus from donating blood?

A. No. While it is true that the AIDS virus can be transmitted through sharing a needle with an infected person, all of the needles that are used in the donation of blood are new and are discarded after a single use. They represent no danger to you in terms of transmitting the AIDS virus.

This question comes up because there are examples of people who received infected blood and eventually developed AIDS. The government now requires every unit of donated blood to be screened for the AIDS virus. Screening measures will nearly eliminate transfusion-related transmission.

This fear of the AIDS virus in association with blood donations has caused blood donations nationwide to drop. The Red Cross is asking a number of people (those who may have had sexual contact with someone in a high-risk category) to refrain from donating blood. Any shortages due to donor exclusion will need to be compensated for by more donations. So, unless you are in a high-risk category, or have had intimate contact with someone who is, you should consider helping the cause by donating blood. You can call your local Red Cross to make arrangements.

29. Q. Who should not donate blood because of the AIDS virus?

    A. The Public Health Service recommends that the following groups refrain voluntarily from donating blood:

    1) Anyone who has had AIDS or one of its signs or symptoms.

    2) Males who have had sex with one or more male partners since 1977.

    3) Males whose sexual partner has had sex with one or more male partners since 1979.

    4) Past or present abusers of intravenous drugs.

    5) Hemophiliacs.

    6) Sexual partners of persons in these groups.

The antibody test currently used to detect the AIDS virus will not always be positive when there is infection. Because of this the Public Health Service is strongly discouraging donations from any individual who thinks he or she might have been exposed to the AIDS virus. Infected blood can pass through this screening and be used to treat patients who may become infected.

Analysis of the first 1.6 million screened blood donations indicate the general public is following these recommendations. Presently there are over 1 million symptomless carriers of the AIDS virus. The Red Cross projects that only 1,600 of its 4 million annual donations this year will indicate infection with the AIDS virus.

30. Q. Have procedures been implemented that will make hemophiliacs safer from contracting the AIDS virus via infected blood products?

    A. Yes. There are two measures which should cut down on the chances of a hemophiliac becoming infected with the AIDS virus through the use of blood products. The first is that as of May 1985 all blood donations are screened for the AIDS virus. This should nearly eliminate infected donations that will be used in the making of blood products. The second precaution is that Factor VIII, a blood product frequently used by hemophiliacs, will be heat treated, which will hopefully kill any AIDS virus that exists within it. However, the effectiveness of heat treatment is controversial.

Although these measures will cut down on AIDS virus infection through the blood supply, AIDS cases will continue to appear in hemophiliacs for a number of years. This is because there is a long (two- to five-year) incubation period in hemophiliacs. Some hemophiliacs infected prior to May 1985 will develop AIDS in the future.

This topic cannot be responsibly covered without mentioning that AIDS virus infection among hemophiliacs is a terrible problem. It is believed that a majority of the nation's hemophiliacs were infected between 1979 and 1984. This group is being carefully monitored for signs and symptoms of AIDS and AIDS-related complex.

31. Q. Are Haitians more susceptible to the AIDS virus than other groups?

A. No. Haitians are neither more nor less susceptible to the AIDS virus than other groups.

This inaccurate supposition arose in late 1981, when, in addition to homosexual men, three distinct groups emerged who also were coming down with AIDS—Haitian-Americans, intravenous drug users, and hemophiliacs.

After the AIDS virus was identified as the cause of AIDS, more careful analysis showed that Haitians who immigrated after 1977 were 40 times more likely to develop AIDS than those who immigrated previous to 1978. From this it was concluded that the cases of AIDS in Haitian-Americans was due to *exposure* to the virus and not increased *susceptibility*. The virus apparently spread throughout the Caribbean, with Haiti one of the first areas in the Western Hemisphere exposed to the AIDS virus.

It is also believed that four characteristics of the Haitian population made it a fertile ground for the AIDS virus to spread. First is the use of unsterilized needles by "picuristes" (healers), which is common. Second, Haiti has a promiscuous homosexual population. Third, Haitian women practice anal sex as a form of birth control. Anal sex is believed to be a practice which facilitates the transmission of the AIDS virus. Fourth, both heterosexual and homosexual prostitution is widely practiced.

Haitian-Americans are no longer specifically identified by the Centers for Disease Control as a high risk group for infection with the AIDS virus.

32. Q. How hardy is the AIDS virus outside the body of an infected host?

A. Unlike most other retroviruses, the AIDS virus can survive outside the body for hours to days. Live virus can be recovered from day-old dried blood (unpublished observations). However, epidemiological studies clearly prove infection results from sexual contact, not environmental exposure. Infection depends on the method of transmission, the quantity of contagion, and the condition of the host at the time of exposure. A number of household cleaning products quickly destroy live AIDS virus.

33. Q. If someone with the AIDS virus visits my house, what steps should I take to see to it that they don't infect someone unknowingly?

A. The first and most obvious answer is to avoid all sexual contact with the infected individual.

The AIDS virus is easy to kill through a variety of ways: exposure to heat, alkalinity (such as a toilet-bowl cleaner), bleach (Clorox, hydrogen peroxide), commercial disinfectant (Lysol), and alcohol. However, even if someone with the AIDS virus visits your home, it is probably unnecessary to clean all surfaces they have had contact with.

On the other hand, if a surface is contaminated with the blood, saliva, urine, tears, or semen of an individual infected with the AIDS virus, it is recommended to clean this surface with a household bleach freshly mixed with water in a 1 to 10 dilution.

Because the virus can be cultured from saliva, it is recommended that you not share utensils with an infected person.

The sharing of toothbrushes and razor blades are possible methods of transmission. If someone visits your house who has the AIDS virus, you should avoid sharing these objects with him or her.

34. Q. What is "safe sex" and how safe is it?

A. When AIDS was first becoming well known in America, it victimized mostly urban male homosexuals. At the time it was not known what caused AIDS, but it was suspected to be a sexually transmitted disease. For this reason, in certain urban areas there were massive public information campaigns aimed at encouraging people to reduce or eliminate casual, anonymous sex. As a secondary suggestion, a set of precautions that came to be known as "safe sex" was described. The campaign for "safe sex" is an implicit admission that people will not cut down on sex entirely, no matter how drastic the possible consequences might be. So "safe sex" is a "next best" alternative.

Simply put, "safe sex" is sex in which no body fluids are exchanged. The AIDS virus has been cultured from the saliva, semen, blood, tears, and urine of infected individuals. Therefore, any practice that involves exposure to these fluids is risky. Safe sex involves no oral-oral, oral-genital, oral-rectal, penile-rectal, or penile-vaginal contact. It involves hugging, touching, massage and masturbation. It is possible but unproven that the use of condoms, diaphragms, and contraceptive jelly may reduce the risk of transmission in oral-penile, penile-rectal, and penile-vaginal sex. For more information, see Chapter 4.

35. **Q.** Do the vaginal secretions of infected women contain AIDS virus?

A. Almost certainly. Vaginal secretions contain large quantities of white blood cells. The AIDS virus permeates the white blood cells of infected individuals. It stands to reason that vaginal secretions of AIDS-virus-positive women contain transmissible virus. Bacteria and yeast have so far hindered investigators' attempts to culture the AIDS virus from vaginal secretions.

36. **Q.** Do condoms help reduce the risk of being infected?

A. Probably. AIDS is a sexually transmitted disease. Condoms have been used for years to help moderate the spread of such sexually transmitted diseases as syphilis and gonorrhea.

The evidence that the use of condoms helps slow the spread of sexually transmitted disease is quite strong. It is likely that the use of condoms will reduce the risk of transmitting the AIDS virus in oral-penile, penile-vaginal, or penile-rectal sex. Please note, though, that kissing is a possible means of transmission, and condoms quite obviously do not eliminate the exchange of saliva.

Condoms do vary in their permeability, making some less effective than others. It should also be noted that condoms may break, in which case they lose all their effectiveness. When condoms are used, the choice of lubricants is crucial. K-Y jelly should be used, since oil-based lubricants such as Vaseline can emulsify and weaken latex condoms.

37. Q. Can contraceptive jelly or diaphragms reduce my risk?

A. Yes. Some contraceptive jellies contain substances such as nonoxynol-9, which is reportedly deadly to the AIDS virus. Contraceptive jelly may help kill virus and thus reduce the risk of transmission in penile-vaginal and penile-rectal sex. The use of diaphragms in addition should also reduce risk.

38. Q. Why is rectal intercourse a high risk sexual activity?

A. Rectal intercourse is especially facilitative for transmitting the AIDS virus. The AIDS virus has been cultured from semen and found to have a very high concentration. During rectal intercourse the lining may be damaged, which will create a direct portal to the bloodstream. In one study approximately one-fifth of male homosexuals reported rectal bleeding after intercourse. A concentrated source of the virus flooding a portal to the bloodstream creates a very high risk situation for transmission.

It is important to recognize that this type of sex is not restricted to homosexual males, and that a wide variety of other sexual activities are recognized as putting individuals at risk, including such seemingly harmless activities as kissing.

39. Q. Is the use of inhalant drugs ("poppers") related to the development of AIDS?

A. Possibly. When AIDS first appeared among homosexual men, researchers investigated the lifestyles of this population to ascertain which, if any, practices might be correlated to the development of AIDS. The use of inhalant drugs, notably amyl and isobutyl nitrite, correlated strongly with reported cases.

For a period of time there was concern that a contaminated batch of drugs was causing the outbreak of AIDS. This was disproved when hemophiliacs, intravenous drug users, and recent Haitian immigrants began appearing with AIDS.

The use of inhalant drugs has proven to correlate with the practice of receptive anal intercourse, which is a sexual practice correlated strongly to both AIDS virus infection and the development of AIDS and ARC.

40. Q. What is the difference between being "exposed to" the AIDS virus and "infected by" the AIDS virus?

A. There are two issues that must be addressed with respect to this question: the medical and the semantic.

Medically, "exposure" could be said to occur if an opportunity for AIDS virus infection took place. This might entail sexual contact or the sharing of a needle with an infected person. If the AIDS virus had an opportunity to gain entrance to a bloodstream and did not, one might say there was "exposure" without "infection." "Infection" takes place when the AIDS virus enters a new bloodstream and genetically invades a T-helper cell.

Semantically, there has been some confusion because some people say "exposed" to soften the impact of the more accurate medical term "infected." At the National Institutes of Health Meeting on Blood Screening on July 31, 1985, an official of the Red Cross was questioned on this point. The topic was notification of donors who had been shown through careful laboratory analysis to have been infected with the AIDS virus. The official was asked if there was a uniform policy on the terminology used in notifying the donor. The official deflected the question to a regional director who indicated that there was no firm policy and that donors with a positive blood test were informed by the use of such ambiguous phrases as "they *may have been exposed,* or *there is a likelihood that they may have been exposed.*" (Emphasis supplied.)

The medical literature on this is unambiguous. An individual with a confirmed positive AIDS virus blood test sequence has been *infected.*

41. Q. If I have been exposed to someone carrying the AIDS virus, can any steps be taken to prevent infection? Specifically, can I take a shot to inactivate the virus?

A. No. There are no "morning after" treatments that can prevent infection from developing if transmission has taken place.

Many people ask this question because of a similar treatment that is given immediately following exposure to hepatitis. When an individual is exposed to hepatitis, there is a shot that effectively prevents infection from taking place. This shot is made from antibodies extracted from the blood of previously infected individuals.

Research is being done on a similar shot (or sequence of shots) for people who have been exposed to the AIDS virus. However, there are tremendous scientific obstacles that stand in the way. Such a shot might potentially cause the disease it is supposed to guard against. It will be years before this could possibly be available.

42. Q. Does general good health for the past several years mean that I am not infected with the AIDS virus?

A. No. One of the reasons that the AIDS virus has been tagged with such labels as the "silent killer" is that most of the people who have been infected do not realize they carry the virus. As a result, they do not know which signs and symptoms indicate AIDS or AIDS-related complex.

Even more disturbing, in terms of the spread of the virus, is that these individuals do not realize that they might infect others. Our current understanding is that 5–20% of infected individuals will develop full-blown AIDS within five years and an additional 25% will develop AIDS-related complex, some of whom will develop full-blown AIDS subsequently.

Even in the individuals who will eventually develop manifestations of the AIDS virus, most will remain symptomless for a period of years. With nearly all infected individuals symptomless for the first year, and more than half still remaining symptomless after five years, it is clear that the population of symptomless infected individuals will continue to grow.

43. Q. Am I safe from the AIDS virus in a city that has not yet had a reported case of AIDS?

A. No. Even in a city in which there has not been a case of AIDS or AIDS-related complex, there may be many symptomless carriers. There are now more than 1 million symptomless people who would be considered indefinitely contagious. Today's sexual reality is that every new partner represents a new chance of infection.

44. Q. Should I stay away from large cities to try and avoid the AIDS virus?

A. Not necessarily. Visiting a large city, even one with a large number of infected people, does not in itself put you at risk. Because the AIDS virus can be transmitted by a finite number of methods, refraining from sex and intravenous drug use protects you from infection in large cities.

This answer deserves elaboration with respect to possible sexual partners. The AIDS virus has infected urban dwellers in large numbers. Cities with large male gay populations have many infected individuals. The virus has undoubtedly made its way into the heterosexual population through bisexual contact, intravenous drug use, and prostitutes.

A "casual" partner from New York City or San Francisco may be more likely to have the AIDS virus than one from, for example, Peoria, Illinois. But trying to devise a "calculus of probability" is somewhat like playing Russian roulette. Probabilities are of negligible consolation to "losers." The best way of guarding against being infected is to abstain from casual, anonymous sex. The next best way is through the practice of "safe sex." (See Chapter 4.)

45. Q. Are multiple sexual partners necessary to catch the AIDS virus?

A. No. Although a number of studies have correlated infected individuals with a large number of sexual partners, this is likely due to the law of probability. To use a simple analogy, every new partner represents a "rolling of the dice." With each new partner representing a possible source of infection, it is not surprising that people with a large number of sexual partners are more likely to have the AIDS virus than those with a small number. This is not due to the cumulative effect of sex with "too many partners." It is due to the increased possibility of having sex with the "wrong partner."

46. Q. Will the current screening procedures for donated blood prevent transfusion-acquired AIDS?

A. Not entirely. It is important to remember that the blood test is a test for antibodies to fight the AIDS virus and not the presence of the virus itself. The presence of antibodies to fight a specific virus are a measure of the body's response to the virus.

There are phases within the course of this disease during which your body may not be producing measurable antibodies to fight the AIDS virus.

The two most likely periods are early in the lifetime of the disease and in its later stages.

In the case of the AIDS virus, most infected individuals will show a positive antibody test between two and eight weeks after infection. However, it has been documented that this period of "latency" can last longer than six months. This means an individual might have been infected by the AIDS virus in the period preceding the blood test (perhaps longer than six months) and not show a positive result on the antibody test.

During the advanced stages of this disease, it is also possible that the body loses its ability to produce antibodies and thus an individual could be infected with the AIDS virus and not show up as a positive on the antibody test. This has been documented in cases of full-blown AIDS.

Data from the first 1.6 million screened donors is encouraging. This procedure will practically eliminate cases of transfusion-related transmission. However, this procedure was only put into effect in May 1985. Due to the long incubation period of the AIDS virus infection, new cases of transfusion-related AIDS will continue to appear for a number of years.

"HOW DO I KNOW IF I'M INFECTED?"

47. Q. Other than taking a blood test, how can I tell whether or not I have been infected with the AIDS virus?

   A. There is no other way to tell. The AIDS virus remains "hidden" in many people without creating any signs or symptoms for one year or more. The only way to tell if you have been infected is to take a blood test. You may have been infected by any sexual partner of the past five years. If you have any reason to suspect you may have been infected, you should consider having your blood tested.

If you have been exhibiting any of the signs or symptoms of either AIDS or AIDS-related complex (detailed on pages 68–69), you should seek medical help.

48. Q. What is the blood test sequence the Red Cross uses in screening blood donations for the AIDS virus?

A. The Red Cross uses a *sequence* of tests in screening blood donations for the AIDS virus. The first test given to a small sample of each donation is called the ELISA. (This is an abbreviation for "enzyme-linked immunosorbent assay.") The ELISA is an extremely sensitive test. Nearly all blood samples that contain the AIDS virus will react positively on the ELISA test. The large majority of blood that is screened will react negatively on the first test, and is passed on for use in transfusion and in the manufacture of blood products.

The ELISA test is so sensitive that it will, in some cases, react positively to blood that is not actually infected with the AIDS virus. For this reason, those samples that are positive on the first ELISA test are again given the ELISA test up to two more times. If the ELISA test is positive two of three times, the risk that it may be infected is considered strong enough so that the donation is not used. If the blood sample reacts positively on the first ELISA test but negatively on two subsequent tests, it is considered uninfected and passed on for use.

Although samples that react positively to two of three ELISA tests are rejected for use, they are not considered definitely infected with the AIDS virus. The Western blot test is then performed.

The Western blot test is so specific that a positive
outcome on blood that has been repeatedly positive on the ELISA test is considered a confirmation
of infection. Only donors with repeatedly positive
ELISA tests that are confirmed by a positive Western blot test are notified that they have been infected. This sequence of tests is now believed to be
quite accurate and is standard in testing for the
AIDS virus.

49. **Q. Is it possible to show up as a positive on the AIDS
virus blood test without having been infected with
the virus?**

   A. Yes, though this is no longer a major medical concern. This is referred to as a "false positive" outcome. The initial test performed in the AIDS virus
blood test sequence is the ELISA test. It is so sensitive that it not only reacts positively to nearly all
infected blood, but in some cases to blood that has
not been infected.

   Early in the history of blood testing for the AIDS
virus, there was a great deal of concern about false
positive outcomes. News that one has been infected is so traumatizing that the possibility of
incorrectly notifying someone should be avoided.

   When the entire AIDS virus blood test *sequence*
is run, it virtually eliminates the possibility of false
positive outcomes.

50. **Q. Where can I get my blood tested for the AIDS
virus?**

   A. There are three possible ways to get your blood
tested. One is as the result of a request by a physician. The second is through donating blood. The
third is at an alternate test site.

   Physicians can order the AIDS virus blood test,
which actually is a blood test sequence. (For details
see question 48.) In general, physicians would order
the test as a result of signs or symptoms suggestive
of AIDS or AIDS-related complex. These include

persistent swollen glands, weight loss, and diarrhea.

The second method of having your blood tested for the AIDS virus is to donate blood. Our nation's blood supply is currently protected by having all blood screened for the AIDS virus. This includes all Red Cross donations and all other regional and local blood-collecting facilities. However, the donation of blood from individuals who suspect they may be infected is vigorously discouraged. The reason for this is the slight chance that the blood test sequence may not identify infected blood. Information on the first 1.6 million pints of donated blood suggests that donors are scrupulously following this suggestion and are not using a blood donation as a surrogate AIDS virus blood test.

In many areas there exists a third method, an alternative site at which an individual can have his or her blood checked for the AIDS virus. As of July 31, 1985, there were 573 such sites in 41 states. Generally an individual needs to call and establish an appointment for a counseling session. Individuals not in the current identified high-risk groups (male homosexuals, intravenous drug users, hemophiliacs, and recent immigrants from the Caribbean and central Africa) have often been discouraged from having the test run, with the possibility of a "false positive" result mentioned. This is a hollow argument because a positive result on the test sequence is clearly indicative of infection.

If an individual arranges an appointment, there is normally a counseling session of half an hour or more that takes place before a decision to have the blood test accepted as valid. Is some cases decisions are not permitted on the first visit and a second visit and counseling session are required.

In spite of these obstacles, a persistent individual who is determined to have his or her blood

tested can get the test done and the results kept
confidential. Early indications do not show the
public taking great advantage of this option. In the
first 10 weeks of such a program in Massachusetts
with eight test sites, only 119 people had the test
done, with 20 infected individuals being identified. August and September saw an explosive increase in alternate-test-site utilization. However,
these facilities will likely identify less than 1% of
our nation's symptomless carriers, in spite of this
important public breakthrough. Epidemiologists
hope that more and more people will be utilizing
these facilities.

If you wish to know where you can get your
blood tested, you may call your local Red Cross,
health department, or any of the organizations
listed in Appendix A (pages 262—267).

**51. Q. What do the tests in the AIDS virus blood test
sequence actually measure?**

A. Both ELISA and the Western blot tests measure the
presence of *antibodies* in the blood that specifically fight the AIDS virus.

When a foreign germ invades the body, the
body's immune system prepares a defense. It produces *antibodies*, which are a protein. They are
weapons used by the body in response to infection.
These antibodies are specific for the type of germ
that it has invaded. For example, if a child has
measles, his blood produces antibodies that are
made to fight the measles.

The tests measure the presence of antibodies
produced specifically to fight the AIDS virus. The
reasoning is that if you have antibodies for the
AIDS virus, you have been infected by the AIDS
virus.

**52. Q. What does a positive or negative result on the
AIDS virus blood test sequence actually mean?**

A. If you are negative, it is safe to say that you are not infected. Although false negative results do exist they are rare enough to be of negligible concern. If you and your sexual partner are both negative on the blood test you can safely pursue a truly monogamous relationship without fear of AIDS virus infection.

If you are positive, it does not necessarily mean that you will develop AIDS. It appears that 5–20% of infected individuals will develop AIDS within five years and an additional 25% will develop AIDS-related complex (ARC), which is described in detail on page 66.

If you are positive, it is safe to say that you have been *infected* (not merely "exposed") with the virus. Dr. Zaki Salahuddin reports that individuals who persistently show antibodies usually harbor cells from which infectious AIDS virus can be recovered.[4] Curran and coworkers also report that the presence of AIDS virus antibody should be considered presumptive evidence of current infection.[5]

Although not all "antibody positive individuals" develop AIDS within five years of infection, they should consider themselves indefinitely infected and infectious. Steps should be taken to follow good general health habits and avoid coinfection with other germs. Safe sex procedures should be rigorously followed to prevent sexual partners from becoming infected, and conceiving children should be indefinitely postponed.

53. Q. What will be done with the results of the test now being used by the Red Cross to screen blood for the AIDS virus?

A. If you have a negative result you will not be informed. If you have a positive result, after the test has been repeated and it is determined that the positive result is not due to laboratory error, you will be informed by the Red Cross. Currently there are three means of notifying donors of a positive result—personal visit, phone call, or certified letter. This notification will take place within three months of the donation.

Donors with a positive test will also be placed on a deferral list of persons who may not give blood. The reason for the deferral will be kept confidential. Only "authorized individuals" will be allowed access to this information. In the future the Red Cross may be required to report positive blood tests for the AIDS virus to the health department, as is now required for some other tests.

The government is currently encouraging safeguards to protect the confidentiality of this information. However, it may in the future be obtainable through the legal process.

54. Q. **Should my physician obtain my approval before ordering the AIDS virus blood test?**

A. Yes. There are other types of blood tests, for which your physician may not necessarily ask for your approval. However, the employment and insurance consequences that could result from a positive blood test for the AIDS virus are so serious that they should be discussed before this test is run. If your physician would like this test on your blood, he or she should discuss beforehand why the test is being done, the significance of a positive or negative determination, and the possible consequences.

55. Q. **Can I refuse to allow my doctor to have my blood tested for the AIDS virus, and what are the possible consequences of such a decision?**

A. Yes. It is within the rights of the individual to refuse any diagnostic test. However, one consequence is that your doctor may refuse to treat you and you will be refused care by the hospital. In agreeing to treat you, the doctor and the hospital are liable for medical consequences that may affect others as a result of your care. It is possible, for example, that if you were infected with the AIDS virus and your doctor did not know this, it may inadvertently be transmitted to others. Those others would then have the legal right to sue your doctor and/or the hospital.

56. Q. Why is the test for the AIDS virus being used to screen blood?

A. Of the first 13,000 cases of AIDS reported to the Centers for Disease Control, 208 were caused by transfusion-related transmission. There is no known way to treat infected blood to safely inactivate the AIDS virus.

57. Q. Is it possible to actually be infected with the AIDS virus and yet show up as a negative on the blood test? Why?

A. Yes. A "false negative" occurs when a person with infected blood does not register positive on the AIDS virus blood test sequence.

The blood test measures antibodies to fight the AIDS virus and not the AIDS virus itself. Immediately after being infected, there is a period of latency. It will usually take from two to eight weeks until an infected individual will begin to show antibody production on the blood test. However, this period of latency can last more than six months.

Because available research indicates up to a 5% false negative result, individuals who believe they may have been infected with the AIDS virus should consider being tested periodically.

"WHAT IF I AM INFECTED?"

58. Q. Am I entitled to receive disability insurance if I am a symptomless carrier of the AIDS virus?

A. Most likely not. Disability insurance pays for replacement of income due to lost work. Since symptomless carriers of the AIDS virus are able to work, they would generally not qualify for disability insurance.

A possible exception is someone in a job in which they are no longer permitted to work due to the possibility that they may infect others in the course of their work. Examples might someday include a doctor, a dentist, or someone who works in food preparation. In such a case, a job change may be necessitated by determination that a person has been infected with the AIDS virus.

Collection of disability insurance in cases such as these may hinge on the wording of the particular policy. It would likely also hinge on the skill of the lawyer trying to collect. This dilemma is merely an example of the sticky, undefined questions posed by the threat of the AIDS virus.

59. Q. **If I am diagnosed as having AIDS-related complex, am I entitled to disability insurance?**

A. Possibly. Disability insurance protects the individual against lost income due to inability to work. AIDS-related complex encompasses a large range of conditions, some of which render an individual unable to work. These conditions include anemia, chronic diarrhea, persistent fever, weight loss, and loss of mental faculties.

The issue of whether an individual with AIDS-related complex qualifies for disability insurance is being approached on a case-by-case basis. Many individuals will likely qualify.

The conditions under which disability insurance will be paid to individuals infected with the AIDS virus are merely one example of the "hornet's nest" of questions being debated with respect to the relationship between private industry and government.

The insurance industry is currently suffering financial stress as a result of having to pay out on various claims resulting from infection with the

AIDS virus. Clearly this risk was unanticipated by the insurance industry. Insurance companies suspect a "loading up" on this type of insurance by people who learn of AIDS virus infection. The monies paid out on these policies was not anticipated in calculating the premiums paid to cover them.

The insurance industry wishes to utilize blood screening as a prerequisite for certain types of policies. For example, in providing medical and disability group insurance in an area where the AIDS virus is extremely prevalent, companies argue for the right to know the numbers (but not necessarily the names) of those infected.

60. Q. If I am diagnosed as having a case of full-blown AIDS, am I entitled to receive disability insurance?

A. Yes. Disability insurance protects the individual against the possibility of losing income due to the inability to work. To receive disability an individual must prove total, permanent inability to work.

Statistics show that 80% of the individuals diagnosed with full-blown AIDS will die within three years of diagnosis, and the other 20% will die within five years of diagnosis. This easily fulfills the requirements for disability insurance.

61. Q. If I am diagnosed as having a case of full-blown AIDS, am I entitled to receive Social Security disability payments?

A. Yes. To qualify for government Social Security disability payments, an individual must have paid into the system and then prove total and permanent inability to do any type of work. A person with full-blown AIDS easily meets these requirements.

Unfortunately, the paperwork involved in receiving government checks typically takes a year or longer. Since the life expectancy of the typical

AIDS patient is 18 months following the diagnosis, a 12-month wait for a Social Security check is much too long.

Fortunately, the Social Security Administration will oftentimes accelerate approval for terminally ill patients. If you have AIDS, you should contact your local Social Security office and petition for early payments. Your physician can help by writing a letter describing the seriousness of your condition. Many hospitals which have handled AIDS patients are familiar with this problem and can help you cut through the bureaucratic red tape. Remember you are dealing with the government, so be persistent. Expect bureaucratic obstacles.

62. Q. **Can people who infect others with the AIDS virus be held legally accountable?**

A. Possibly. Prudential Insurance recently made an out-of-court settlement of $25,000 with a woman who had contracted genital herpes from one of its homeowner policyholders. The woman had consented to having sexual relations with the man but had not "consented" to catch genital herpes from him. Prudential agreed to pay the woman the maximum possible benefit from that particular policy. Although this does not represent legal precedent, it provides an early report of a developing legal issue.

Some politically extreme individuals are calling the willing spread of AIDS virus infection a grounds for involuntary manslaughter. Conversation such as this can be currently categorized as "rhetoric" rather than a serious legislative proposal.

It will be nearly impossible to apply civil or criminal statutes on a practical basis. Due to the long dormancy of the virus, it would be necessary to prove that the infected individual was an exclusive sexual partner for a considerable period of time. Cases such as these will crop up, but not in great numbers. Certainly an infected individual who practices "unsafe sex" is demonstrating reckless disregard for his or her partner. Such an individual needs reeducation and counseling, and in some cases even civil restraint.

63. Q. If I have the AIDS virus, can I be quarantined?

A. Not at present. One interesting *de facto* example came in New Haven, Connecticut. A prostitute with full-blown AIDS was released from a hospital and had returned to work as a streetwalker. She represented a threat to the public health, but city officials did not want to try and invoke quarantine powers. She was arrested on prostitution and drug possession charges and eventually died in jail. Her case was never tried on civil liberties grounds.

At times in the past, our government has utilized quarantine powers to stop the spread of deadly infectious disease. Legal justification for this is rooted in the notion that one proper role of government is to protect the innocent against unanticipated catastrophe. The doctrine of *parens patriae* ("state as father") is the basis for laws against suicide and euthanasia. There is ample precedent for a range of government interventions designed to protect the public health, of which quarantine is the most severe.

The British government has established quarantine powers within the Public Health Ministry to help curb the spread of the AIDS virus. The British have given broad powers to local magistrates to quarantine individuals who are willingly infecting others.

This is precisely the type of governmental intervention most feared by those in the identified high-risk groups in America. Male homosexuals in particular have expressed concern about an erosion of civil liberties which could lead to such mea-

sures as quarantine. Discussions of quarantine
make for dramatic headlines but have little practical value in slowing the spread of the AIDS virus
infection. (See pages 226–230.)

64. Q. **Other than quarantine, what methods has government used in the past to prevent the spread of infectious disease?**

A. One method is to utilize a blood test as a screening
device. The military screens for venereal disease in
its candidates. Applicants determined to be infected with venereal disease are treated before
being allowed to join the armed forces.

A similar procedure is performed on couples
applying for a marriage license in any state. If the
AIDS virus blood test were used as a marital
screen it would be a more dramatic step. Unlike
syphilis, there is no treatment for AIDS virus infection. Thus a screen would prevent, not merely
delay, marriage or joining the military.

A second method is to make a disease reportable. (Full-blown AIDS is reportable in 45 states,
and AIDS virus infection will be reportable in
Colorado starting October 30, 1985.) Any health
care professional diagnosing a reportable disease
must send a form to the local health department
which may by state law require the patient's name
and address, the doctor's name, and in some cases
other medical information. This can be used for
follow-up and for gathering statistical data. A more
dramatic intervention is the practice of contact
tracing. In this, individuals with a reportable sexually transmissible disease are requested to provide information about recent sexual contacts so
that these people may be alerted. Civil penalties
are usually attached to withholding information,
but these are difficult to enforce.

More dramatic than contact tracing is the mechanism of declaring a "health hold" order. This is issued by an authorized official to an individual, requiring him to cooperate with examination or treatment. Violation of a health hold order can result in an individual being involuntarily held either if the person does not cooperate or there is reasonable suspicion that he or she may not cooperate. Health hold orders are often issued when a hospital is treating an individual who is being held for a sexual crime.

Finally, there is a precedent for involuntary immunization of specific high risk groups. There have been examples of certain populations being immunized, notably school children and military personnel going to an area in which there is tropical disease. Immunization laws usually require that there be a provable risk to a specific population before involuntary immunization is permitted. This may become a legal issue if a vaccine for the AIDS virus is developed in the future.

65. Q. **If the AIDS threat continues to grow, what would likely be the sequence of steps government would take to prevent the spread of infection?**

A. The question of national control of sexually transmitted disease has been approached academically by legal scholar Donald C. Bross in the medical text *Sexually Transmitted Diseases.*[6] His three-step plan included the following:

PHASE I
1) Enact enabling legislation to state the basic purposes, authority and limitations of public health efforts to control sexually transmitted diseases.
2) Authorize epidemiological studies by gathering confidential data to determine incidence and prevalence of sexually transmitted diseases in each sector of the population.

PHASE II

3) Based on prior experiences and data gathered in Phase I, establish public clinics, confidential sexually-transmitted-disease special physicians, or other preferred programs of intervention. Enact appropriate licensing legislation.

4) Require reporting of sexually transmitted disease by all health care professionals.

5) Authorize contact tracing and health hold orders based on reasonable suspicion of exposure. Expressly authorize health holds for specific groups, such as detained prostitutes where appropriate.

PHASE III

6) Authorize physical examinations on an involuntary basis, if this was not done previously.

7) Permit screening of epidemiologically documented high-risk groups. Note that this permits screening even when there is no exposure on which to form a basis for evaluation. Designate high-risk groups as appropriate.

8) Consider authorizing large-scale screening to issuance of identity cards as part of a major crackdown, if resources are available and prevalence figures warrant an effort of this degree.

66. **Q. What is full-blown acquired immune deficiency syndrome?**

A. To be diagnosed as having "full-blown AIDS" a person has to fulfill the criteria defined by the Centers for Disease Control for the acquired immune deficiency syndrome. The term "full-blown" AIDS is often used to designate that a person has, in fact, had at least one life-threatening opportunistic infection or Kaposi's sarcoma, and not one of the non-life-threatening manifestations of the AIDS virus, such as seen in AIDS-related complex patients.

Statistics show that 80% of the people diagnosed

as having "full-blown" AIDS will die within three years of the diagnosis, and the rest will die within five years. Full-blown AIDS is the end-state of infection with the AIDS virus and, as defined here, provides a useful, unambiguous reference point for clinical and epidemiologic study. (See Appendixes B and C, pages 268–270.)

67. Q. **How many cases of full-blown AIDS have been diagnosed so far? What can be expected through 1986?**

A. As of September 23, 1985, there were 13,216 adult AIDS cases reported in the United States. It is expected that there will be more than 17,000 additional cases reported in 1986.

68. Q. **What is an "opportunistic infection"?**

A. There are many germs in the environment that, under normal circumstances, can easily be rendered harmless by the immune system. However, with a damaged immune system, characteristic of people who have been attacked by the AIDS virus, these normally harmless germs can become killers.

This is why AIDS is referred to as a "syndrome." The AIDS virus attacks the immune system (the body's system for fighting infection), allowing various germs to infect and possibly kill. These germs include viruses, fungi, bacteria, and protozoa.

The most common opportunistic infection in AIDS patients at diagnosis is *Pneumocystis carinii*, which causes an often fatal pneumonia. Other germs that attack AIDS patients include *Toxoplasma gondii*, *Cryptosporidium*, *Candida* species, *Cryptococcus neoformans*, *Mycobacterium avium-intracellularie*, *Mycobacterium tuberculosis*, cytomegalovirus, Herpes simplex virus, herpes zoster virus, Epstein-Barr virus, and many others.

69. Q. **What is AIDS-related complex, and how serious is it?**

A. AIDS-related complex (ARC) is a constellation of signs and symptoms manifested by persons who have been infected with the AIDS virus. These manifestations may include generalized swollen glands for greater than three months, recurrent fever greater than 100°F. for at least three months, weight loss greater than 10% of body weight or 15 pounds, chronic diarrhea, fatigue, night sweats, and a variety of laboratory abnormalities.

The line that separates AIDS-related complex from full-blown AIDS is indistinct. It can be said that AIDS-related complex is generally characterized by non-life-threatening conditions. In some cases of ARC, patients will develop life-threatening infections such as *Pneumocystis carinii* or Kaposi's sarcoma (a rare skin cancer). These patients are then classified as having full-blown AIDS. Individuals with ARC are generally more infectious than those with AIDS.

It is clear that while AIDS-related complex is, in itself, not usually life threatening, a percentage of people with ARC will develop full-blown AIDS. The exact percentage that will progress to full-blown AIDS is a matter of dispute. Some physicians feel that a large percentage of people with ARC will eventually develop full-blown AIDS.

70. Q. What is "pre-AIDS" (pre–acquired immune deficiency syndrome)?

A. "Pre-AIDS" is a term used to describe persons with some form of AIDS-related complex who will most likely go on to develop the full-blown acquired immune deficiency syndrome. It has been observed that some of the people with AIDS-related complex will develop AIDS. It is currently not known what percentage of ARC people will eventually develop AIDS. It is also not known what cofactors make it more or less likely for a patient with ARC to develop full-blown AIDS. For these reasons, the term "pre-AIDS" should be avoided.

71. Q. What is chronic lymphadenopathy syndrome and how is it related to AIDS?

A. Chronic lymphadenopathy syndrome is one of the possible medical complications collectively known as AIDS-related complex (ARC). It is, in simple terms, a persistent case of swollen glands. People with chronic lymphadenopathy syndrome have large swollen glands in two or more areas other than the groin for a period of at least three months.

A physician will diagnose lymphadenopathy syndrome if there are no other current illnesses or drug use known to cause swollen glands. To confirm diagnosis, a doctor will remove a small piece of the gland and investigate it under the microscope for a characteristic appearance.

At least 10% of the patients who have chronic lymphadenopathy syndrome will progress to full-blown AIDS. With lymphadenopathy syndrome, patients may also be more likely to eventually develop lymphoma, or cancer of the glands.

72. Q. Does the AIDS virus cause cancer?

A. Yes. The AIDS virus has been associated with certain cancers, including Kaposi's sarcoma, lymphoma, and Hodgkin's disease. How the virus causes these cancers is unknown. There is discussion within the medical community as to whether this is a direct or indirect effect.

Prevailing opinion is that "cofactors" are involved, including common viral infections such as mononucleosis cytomegalovirus or papillomavirus, and factors contributing to cell growth. It is clear that when these cofactors appear in association with the AIDS virus, they are very deadly.

Current information only describes the natural history of the diseases observed with AIDS since its emergence here 5 years ago. A 10-, 15-, or 20-year natural history will show correlation with other types of cancer.

The AIDS virus is a member of the retrovirus family. A retrovirus (HTLV-I) was the first established infectious cause of cancer, specifically a certain form of leukemia. This provided an important clue to Dr. Robert Gallo in his search for the cause of AIDS at the National Cancer Institute. The period of dormancy of HTLV-I virus is quite long. Typically, a 15- to 20-year time period elapses between infection and the onset of leukemia. The similarities already apparent with retrovirus family members suggest the sobering possibility that the medical future for AIDS-virus-positive people is even dimmer than current data would imply.

Research on the interactions of the AIDS virus and cancer will certainly help develop further medical interventions on the cancer front.

73. **Q. What are some of the physical indications that I may be developing AIDS or ARC?**

   A. These are some of the signs and symptoms to look for:

    1) Skin—Purple or reddish blotches or bumps (raised or flat, usually painless) may appear on the skin or on the lining of the mouth or rectum. This may indicate Kaposi's sarcoma. Other changes may include scaling along the hairline, generalized darkening of the skin, and a patchy loss of hair. Individuals who have been previously infected by herpes may have more frequent and painful recurrences.

    2) Eyes—There may be a deterioration in vision and the appearance of spots in front of the eyes.

    3) Blood and Glands—There may be easy bruising and fluctuating swelling of the glands in the neck, underarm, or groin area, associated with

aching discomfort. There may also be enlargement of the spleen.

4) Digestive Tract—There may be an overgrowth of yeast throughout the digestive tract. This may produce "cheesy" white deposits in the mouth (oral thrush), dry mouth, sore throat, and painful swallowing. Watery diarrhea is among the most frequent complications of infection with the AIDS virus. Pain during a bowel movement may be caused by an AIDS-related inflammation of the rectum. Rectal bleeding may also occur.

5) Respiratory System—A persistent or dry cough (no phlegm) with or without shortness of breath (not apparently from smoking). There is also an increased chance of developing bacterial infections, such as bronchitis or pneumonia, producing a cough with phlegm.

6) Musculoskeletal System—There may be diffuse aches and pains of the muscles and joints, possibly with fever.

7) Neurological System—There may be a persistent headache, loss of memory, difficulty walking, confusion, irrational behavior, personality change, or seizure. Strength and sensation may be affected in different parts of the body.

8) General Effects—Extreme fatigue, loss of interests, night sweats, sweating, loss of libido, withdrawal and other signs of depression, fever, and rapid weight loss for no apparent reason.

If any of these symptoms or signs appear, it does not necessarily mean that an individual is developing either AIDS or ARC. But an infected individual or an individual at risk who begins showing any of the above signs or symptoms should seek medical evaluation and professional advice.

74. Q. If I am infected, what steps should I take to protect others?

A. The Food and Drug Administration (FDA) in March 1985 made these recommendations to infected individuals:

1) The prognosis for an individual infected with the AIDS virus over the long term is not known. However, data available from studies conducted among homosexual men indicate that most persons will remain infected.

2) Although symptomless, these individuals may transmit the AIDS virus to others. Regular medical evaluation and follow-up is advised, especially for individuals who develop signs or symptoms suggestive of AIDS.

3) Refrain from donating blood, plasma, body organs, other tissues, or sperm.

4) There is a risk of infecting others by sexual intercourse, sharing of needles, and, possibly, exposure of others to saliva through oral-genital contact or intimate kissing. The efficacy of condoms in preventing infection with the AIDS virus is unproven, but the consistent use of them may reduce transmission.

5) Toothbrushes, razors, or other implements that could become contaminated with blood should not be shared.

6) Women with a positive test, or women whose sexual partner is positive, are themselves at increased risk of acquiring AIDS. If they become pregnant, their offspring are also at increased risk of acquiring AIDS.

7) After accidents resulting in bleeding, contaminated surfaces should be cleaned with household bleach freshly diluted 1 to 10 in water.

8) Devices that have punctured the skin, such as hypodermic and acupuncture needles, should be steam sterilized by autoclave before reuse or safely discarded. Whenever possible, disposable needles and equipment should

be used.

9) When seeking medical or dental care of inter-current illness, these persons should inform those responsible for their care of the status so that appropriate evaluation can be undertaken and precautions taken to prevent transmission to others.

10) Testing for the AIDS virus should be offered to persons who may have been infected as a result of their contact with AIDS virus positive individuals (e.g., sexual partners, persons with whom needles have been shared, infants born to seropositive mothers).

75. Q. If I am infected with the AIDS virus, should I tell a potential sexual partner?

A. Emphatically *yes*. The AIDS virus is more than an "inconvenience" or a "temporary embarrassment." It cannot be treated by one visit to the public health department or one shot of penicillin. Once it infects someone, it remains inside that person apparently for an entire lifetime. As long as it is inside an individual, it is potentially deadly.

The "range of infectivity" of the AIDS virus is unknown. The AIDS virus may prove to have variable infectivity, as does, for example, the herpes virus. When the herpes virus is in a period of dormancy (remission), it cannot be transmitted. It is possible that the AIDS virus has a similar pattern. However, until this is known and can be accurately predicted, infected individuals should abstain from sex. A "second best" solution is the practice of "safe sex."

The only hope for slowing the spread of the deadly AIDS virus is a widespread voluntary revision of sexual habits. Someone who knowingly and willingly infects an unsuspecting partner could be committing murder. Someone who unknowingly infects an unsuspecting partner could be committing involuntary manslaughter.

76. Q. **If I am infected with the AIDS virus, can I transmit the virus to my spouse or children?**

A. Yes. The AIDS virus can be transmitted sexually, through the blood, from mother to infant, and through the sharing of infected needles (as with intravenous drug users). Husband and wife can transmit the virus to one another through sexual contact. An infected woman can transmit it to her infant, either through the placenta or through infected milk. Research indicates that infected, pregnant women are at increased risk for developing AIDS.

It is unlikely that the AIDS virus can be transmitted to children through normal household contact or by hugging or touching. If it is determined that either parent is infected, FDA recommendations should be followed to prevent transmission of the AIDS virus. (See question 74.)

77. Q. **If I am pregnant and find out I have the AIDS virus, should I abort the fetus?**

A. This is a very difficult question because of the relative lack of information.

It has been established that a mother who carries the virus with no symptoms of AIDS or ARC can transmit the disease to her unborn infant. In one study of 16 mothers who developed either AIDS or ARC, all but 1 was clinically well at the time of the birth of her first infected child. Ten of the 16 developed AIDS or ARC within a 30-month period. Six of 11 mothers who underwent a subsequent pregnancy developed clinical disease (AIDS or ARC) during that pregnancy.

It appears that mothers are the source of infection in their infants, that infectivity can persist for a prolonged period of time, and that mothers themselves are at risk (probably increased risk) for

AIDS or ARC. However, since five mothers delivered six infants subsequently who are clinically and immunologically normal, there is also evidence that infectivity is variable.

For this reason, if you are planning a pregnancy, you should consider having your blood and your spouse's blood checked for the AIDS virus. If it is determined that either of you has the virus, you should delay the pregnancy indefinitely. If the pregnancy is already in progress, it is recommended you seek qualified medical advice to learn the state of research on this question. Personal and religious counseling may provide worthwhile advice.

78. Q. Does everyone who develops full-blown AIDS die as a result of the syndrome?

A. Yes. The average life expectancy for someone diagnosed with AIDS is 18 months. Eighty percent of those diagnosed with full-blown AIDS die within three years of diagnosis, and the other 20% die within five years.

79. Q. If I am infected with the AIDS virus what are the chances I will develop AIDS or ARC?

A. It is critically important to understand that identification of the presence of the AIDS virus does not necessarily mean you will develop AIDS. Available data suggest that there is better than a 50 percent chance you will not have any manifestations of AIDS or AIDS-related complex within five years of infection.

Only a percentage of those who contract the AIDS virus will develop AIDS within the first five years. Indications are that at least 5% and perhaps 20% or more will develop AIDS within five years of infection. An additional 25% will develop some form of AIDS-related complex, or ARC. ARC can take a number of forms, including swollen glands, persistent fever, weight loss, and diarrhea. Some of those who develop AIDS-related complex will develop AIDS.

Beyond the first five years, it is at this point impossible to project. It could be that if you remain symptomless beyond a certain point, the risk of developing AIDS or ARC decreases. It could be that the AIDS virus can be "triggered" later in life by a significant medical event or chronic condition (such as pregnancy, gallbladder surgery, or diabetes). The long-range connection between the AIDS virus and a variety of blood malignancies, leukemia, and lymphoma is under current investigation. Since the transmission pattern has not been fully described, symptomless people with the AIDS virus should consider themselves infectious.

Because the disease is relatively new, it is not known what the consequences of infection are beyond five years. It *does* appear that the virus stays in the body indefinitely, and that as long as it is in the body there exists the potential to infect others.

80. Q. **What are "cofactors" and what is their relationship to the development of AIDS?**

A. The AIDS virus has a period of dormancy in infected individuals. It will not create symptoms for a period which can last at least six months and can be longer than five years. It has been suggested this period of dormancy is ended (and a period of active replication begun) in many cases by the "triggering" effect of "cofactors."

Cofactors may be any of a series of independent influences which combine with the AIDS virus during the course of an individual's illness. Genetic variation has been suggested as one possible cofactor. Environmental conditions have also been suggested as a cofactor. These include poor sanitation, malnutrition, and overall poor health habits. Drugs (both prescription and illicit) have also been mentioned as possible cofactors for the variety of illnesses that are related to AIDS virus infection.

Probably the most important cofactors will prove to be various germs which cause intercurrent illnesses. One example of this is the Epstein-Barr virus, which is the cause of mononucleosis. When this is combined with the AIDS virus, it seems to be associated with unusual forms of lymphoma, or cancer of the glands. Kaposi's sarcoma, a skin cancer that is often part of full-blown AIDS, seems to appear more commonly in individuals who have been infected with cytomegalovirus.

Cofactors are an important part of the total makeup of the various outcomes of the AIDS virus. Individuals who remain symptomless for more than five years may have long-range medical complications as a result of their infection with the AIDS virus. It is possible that Rock Hudson's heart surgery in 1981 helped "trigger" the replication of the AIDS virus, leading to full-blown AIDS.

Some suggest that cofactors are *necessary* for the AIDS virus to attack the immune system and develop into ARC or AIDS. The validity of this theory is seriously challenged by individuals who have developed AIDS without any apparent cofactors.

Cofactors have also been suggested in relation to transmission of the AIDS virus. Cofactors may increase or decrease an individual's susceptibility to AIDS virus infection. Much attention is being focused on the route of transmission, dose of contagion, and the general health at the time of exposure. (See pages 102–103.)

81. Q. **Could infection by more than one variant of the AIDS virus be an important cofactor leading to the development of AIDS?**

A. Yes. Dr. Robert Gallo has isolated 18 different variants of the AIDS virus and has evidence indicating there may be more. It is possible that some variants are more virulent than others. If this is true, it would mean that individuals infected with a less virulent variant would have a smaller likelihood of developing AIDS or ARC.

Individuals who are infected with the AIDS virus should observe precautions so that they are not infected by another variant. By introducing a second variant, they run the risk that it is more virulent either by itself or in concert with the variant with which they are already infected.

Many studies indicate that promiscuity correlates with the development of AIDS. This may be due to the fact that promiscuous individuals are more likely to become infected to begin with. It is also possible that individuals who become infected with multiple variants of the AIDS virus are more likely to develop AIDS.

The fact that multiple variants of the AIDS virus exist is one of the obstacles to the development of an effective vaccine.

82. Q. **Is there any difference in the average incubation period for AIDS according to the method of transmission?**

A. Yes. Dr. Anthony Fauci, one of the leading clinical investigators on AIDS in the country, has done the initial work in this area. The "incubation period" (also referred to as "dormancy") is the period from infection with the AIDS virus to the development of clinical manifestations of ARC or AIDS.

Dr. Fauci has calculated that people infected as a result of sexual contact will show the first signs in approximately 12 to 14 months, people infected by a contaminated needle in two years, transfusion recipients and hemophiliacs in two to five years, and infants in a matter of months.

83. Q. **What complications are typical of AIDS, and what can be done to treat them?**

A. A wide variety of complications can occur while a person has acquired immune deficiency syndrome. A common condition among AIDS patients is Kaposi's sarcoma, a previously rare type of skin cancer. Other conditions typical of AIDS include neurological deterioration, swollen glands, persistent fever, unintentional weight loss, diarrhea, and night sweats.

AIDS patients are subject to attack from a number of germs previously seen only infecting cancer-chemotherapy and organ-transplant patients. Physicians have tried a number of agents in attempting to combat the multiple infections characteristic of the syndrome. Nothing has been found to be consistently effective, although some new drugs show promise. The *real* problem is the underlying immune deficiency. What typically happens is that either the treated infections recur or other equally life-threatening infections take place.

There is chemotherapy available which slows down the progression of Kaposi's sarcoma. However, this therapy further damages the immune system, and patients with Kaposi's sarcoma typically die of some type of infection.

84. Q. **What therapy is there on the horizon for treating AIDS?**

A. The only real hope for a cure is to attack and destroy the virus itself. This is particularly difficult because the AIDS virus hides itself within the genes of the host. Some of the drugs being investigated attempt to block the integration of the virus into the genetic structure, while others attempt to block its reemergence from the gene. There is no drug on the horizon that can totally destroy all of the AIDS virus material in the body of an infected individual.

Antiviral Agents:

l) *Suramin*—has proven effectiveness *in vitro* (in

a test tube) at inhibiting replication of the virus once it has entered a host. The mechanics by which it inhibits replication are currently unknown. Preliminary work with humans is proceeding at the National Institutes of Health (Washington, D.C.) and the Claude Bernard Hospital (Paris). A new series of trials is beginning with patients who have AIDS, ARC, or Kaposi's sarcoma at the University of California at San Francisco, the University of California at Los Angeles, the M. D. Anderson Hospital and Tumor Center (Houston), Beth Israel Hospital (New York), the New England Deaconess Hospital (Boston), and the Walter Reed Army Institute of Research (Washington, D.C.)

2) *HPA-23*—This drug has recently received a great deal of public attention because of its use by Rock Hudson. HPA-23 is an agent that is being tried extensively in France and more recently in the United States. It has been shown to work in the test tube, at the Hospital La Pitié Salpetrière in France. HPA-23 has been tried on patients with both AIDS and ARC. It has been shown to inhibit replication of the AIDS virus. However, *it has not been shown to correlate to clinical improvement.* When treatments of HPA-23 are withdrawn, replication of the virus resumes. Additionally, there are several worrisome side effects, notably liver damage, which may limit its serious value as a long-term intervention.

3) *Phosphonoformate*—Phosphonoformate has been effective in the test tube at the Harvard Medical School. It is untested in humans.

4) *Ribavirin*—Ribavirin also has been shown to be effective in a test tube. It will be used in human trials in patients with AIDS-related

complex at Cornell Medical College in New York City.

5) *Ansamycin LM427*—Ansamycin LM427 has been shown to be effective in the test tube in work at the Centers for Disease Control in Atlanta. It has not been tested in humans.

6) *Recombinant Alpha Interferon*—Recombinant alpha interferon received adverse publicity because it proved ineffective when used later in the course of disease with AIDS patients. It has shown to be effective in the test tube and may prove to be somewhat effective if it is used closer to the time of infection. Clinical trials in patients with AIDS-related complex is planned at Harvard.

Immune Modulators

There is another group of drugs under investigation that do not attack the AIDS virus itself. Rather, they help strengthen the immune system. These drugs include interleukin-2, isoprinosine, gamma interferon, levamisole, IMREG 1, and various thymic humoral factors. Many of these do give a boost to the immune system. These drugs were actively discussed at the International Conference on AIDS in Atlanta. The consensus was that the overall effect of these interventions was judged inadequate.

These are some of the drug treatments being investigated to try and provide relief in AIDS and ARC patients. Because of the large scientific obstacles that stand in the way and the cautious pace at which medical science proceeds, it does not seem realistic to anticipate a breakthrough in the near future. But work is clearly proceeding as quickly as science and research funding will permit.

Dr. Anthony Fauci, at the National Institutes of Health, had this to say in November 1984:

We know a lot about the acquired immune deficiency syndrome and the causative agent. However, the problem is by no means solved, and, in fact, the solution is not even in sight…at present there is no effective preventative or treatment regimen for the virus itself.

Dr. Martin S. Hirsch, associate professor of medicine of the Harvard Medical School, had this to say in April 1985:

We have a long way to go before AIDS is either preventable or treatable, but the first steps have been taken. I think we're on our way.

"HOW DOES AIDS AFFECT EVERYONE?"

85. Q. Isn't it basically a small number of groups who should be concerned about the spread of the AIDS virus? Aren't "normal people" basically safe?

A. No. Every American should be concerned. During 1979, the AIDS virus was infecting an average of 7 people per day, many of them male homosexuals. Today the AIDS virus is infecting more than 1,000 people per day, including many heterosexuals.

Even an individual who enjoys a monogamous relationship with an uninfected partner should be concerned about the spread of the AIDS virus. In dollars and cents alone, AIDS is going to be very costly for our nation. It currently costs $140,000 in immediate outlays to pay for medical costs of AIDS patients. It is conceivable that by the end of the decade as many as 1 million Americans will have AIDS, which would cost our nation more than $100 billion in direct outlays alone.

The challenge of the AIDS crisis cuts across political lines. It involves philosophical and practical questions of civil liberties, medical ethics, marriage licensing, and a wide range of questions that will redefine the relationship between the individual and the government. No American should forfeit his or her right to participate in this vital national debate that is upon us.

86. Q. How serious a problem is AIDS in infants and children?

A. "Pediatric AIDS" is a growing problem. The first cases of pediatric AIDS were reported in 1982. As of September 23, 1985, there were 185 cases reported from 22 states.

It is estimated that in New York City alone there are an average of two children born each day to mothers with AIDS virus infection. Infants can be infected by the mother either directly, through the placenta, or indirectly, via infected milk. Infants and children have also been infected by contaminated transfusions and blood products.

One example of the latter is Ryan White, a 13-year-old from Kokomo, Indiana, who has AIDS. Ryan is a hemophiliac who was infected by contaminated blood products. Recent federal procedures should practically eliminate infection by blood, blood products and donated organs. However there is an incubation period of two to five years for AIDS caused by this kind of transmission. There will be cases appearing over the next several years in which infection took place prior to the implementation of screening procedures (in May 1985).

87. Q. Is AIDS a divine retribution for the promiscuity of modern times?

A. This clearly is a question that no one can answer authoritatively, though it is being debated fervently. There are a few observations on this subject that are worth making.

Promiscuity has been a part of civilized culture for as long as history has been recorded. It has survived wars, famine, political upheaval, the industrial revolution, and the communications revolution. It is difficult to measure objectively over the sweep of history. Who can say, for example, that extramarital sex is more or less prevalent now than in Victorian England? Just as promiscuity has always been present, so have there been a ready band of "doomsday adventists" proclaiming that "the end is near."

It is also clear that modern advances in contraception facilitated promiscuous lifestyles. With the advent of the birth control pill, women have relative control over the specter of an unwanted pregnancy. While it is hard to say definitely whether or not promiscuity in general has increased over the last two decades, it certainly has become less clandestine. Unmarried couples live together today with far less constraint and social ostracism than a few decades ago.

This openness about promiscuity has been challenged by the fear of sexually transmitted disease. When herpes was widely publicized as a threat in the middle 1970s, some people reassessed their choices—particularly by cutting down on casual, anonymous sex.

The threat that the AIDS virus represents certainly should cause a major revision of how people view sexual mores. This will not necessarily be a reassessment on moral or religious grounds—rather, on practical grounds. With every new sexual partner representing the possibility of deadly infection, it would not be surprising to see in the heterosexual world what has already been observed in the male homosexual world—a major revision in lifestyle.

88. Q. If AIDS is supposed to be a "homosexual disease" why does it not affect female homosexuals (lesbians)?

A. AIDS has affected male homosexuals in large

numbers. In contrast, very few female homosexuals (lesbians) have been infected with the virus through sexual contact. While the AIDS virus can be transmitted sexually, it is not a "homosexual disease" any more than herpes is a "heterosexual disease."

A sexually transmitted disease needs a "portal of entry" in order to affect a group. For example, if half a dozen promiscuous students returned to a college campus carrying the virus in the fall, the virus would have achieved a "portal of entry" to that campus.

The AIDS virus has not apparently achieved a significant "portal of entry" to the female homosexual (lesbian) community. In this way, the AIDS virus fits the pattern of other sexually transmitted diseases. The lesbian community has one of the lowest rates of infection of sexually transmitted disease of all distinct populations. This is believed to be due to a lack of promiscuity among lesbians.

This fact demonstrates conclusively that AIDS is *not* a "homosexual" disease. It is a virus that can be sexually transmitted, and can be transmitted through both heterosexual and homosexual contact.

89. Q. Since it is possible for false positive blood test results to occur, isn't it wrong to stigmatize people on the basis of blood results?

A. Much has been made about the stigmatizing effects of false positive results. Fortunately, the blood test sequence currently used to identify AIDS virus infection has been verified as both highly sensitive and highly specific. If blood proves positive on all three aspects of the sequence, it correctly identifies infection in 99% of the cases. This accuracy is much greater than with many other tests whose validity is widely accepted, such as the EKG utilized to determine insurability.

Advocates of high-risk groups (of which homo-

sexuals are currently the most politically organized) will continue to use the "false positive argument." Many of the examples they cite are from a
time in which the blood test sequence was not as
reliable as it is today. Gay-rights advocates justifiably fear the possible consequences that may result
from identification of AIDS virus infection. Housing restrictions, loss of employment or insurance,
prosecution for violation of sodomy statutes, and
quarantining of infected persons have all been
mentioned.

Since these concerns involve basic civil liberties,
they defy simple solution. Because the AIDS virus
blood test sequence is now so accurate these questions can be properly debated on their own merits
and not with the obsolete grounds of false positive
results.

90. Q. Is AIDS a problem in the prison system?

A. Yes. AIDS cases in prison are rapidly increasing.
There is widespread homosexual contact and drug
use among prisoners, yet little is generally done to
protect inmates against AIDS virus infection. The
problem is compounded by rules in many prisons
which forbid sex and make condoms unavailable.
Preventive procedures, notably "safe sex," may
lessen the future cost of caring for AIDS cases in
prison hospitals and will also help prevent the
eventuality of releasing thousands of infected individuals whose terms expire or who earn parole.

**91. Q. Is the AIDS virus blood test required for a mar-
riage license in any state?**

A. No. The blood test that is given as a requirement for
marriage is a test for syphilis. If either of the applicants has a blood test indicating past infection by
syphilis, the license is denied until that individual
is treated by the health department or can prove
previous treatment. The reasoning behind this is
protection of the public health and prevention of
the spread of syphilis.

It is likely that the AIDS virus is a more common infection in the American population than is syphilis. Furthermore, it is quite clear that the AIDS virus can be transmitted heterosexually and from mother to infant. There are examples of symptomless parents bearing children who develop AIDS or AIDS-related complex. In New York City alone an average of two babies per day are born with the AIDS virus. It is not surprising, therefore, to hear voices clamoring for the consideration of the drastic step of having the AIDS virus test be a marital screen. In June 1985, the *Journal of the American Medical Association* came out in an editorial recommending consideration of this step.

It is clear this would be a drastic action. Unlike syphilis, which can be treated by the public health department, the AIDS virus cannot be killed by any known means. A marital screening for the AIDS virus would not mean delaying a marriage. It would mean preventing it. (See pages 223–224.)

92. Q. **Does the military plan to use the AIDS virus blood test to screen recruits?**

A. Yes. In a decision announced by the armed services on August 30, 1985, as of October 1985, all recruits are being screened for the AIDS virus. Infected individuals would be barred from entering the military. This is especially significant because it is the first example of the use of the blood test to restrict employment.

One reason the military became concerned about AIDS virus infection was the development of smallpox in one of its recruits. In May a 19-year-old presumed to be healthy was injected with a live smallpox vaccine and subsequently developed smallpox. Army physicians found that he was suffering immune system damage as a result of a replicative attack by the AIDS virus.

Army Doctor Edmund Tramount, speaking before the Armed Forces Epidemiological Board on

August 9, said that the armed forces had a justifiable reason to screen for AIDS virus infection. He cited the example of an immune suppressed soldier sent to disease-prone areas and being unable to function properly. In its decision to reject for induction all infected individuals, the military has taken a much broader approach. The military will also screen all 2.1 million active-duty personnel.

93. Q. Is AIDS currently a "reportable" disease?

A. Yes. This means county and state health departments must be notified upon diagnosis of the disease in any individual. Reportable diseases are identified by the Centers for Disease Control in Atlanta. Each disease is defined by what is known as a surveillance definition. This is to standardize reporting on the disease, so that scientists are able to compare, as the saying goes, "apples with apples." AIDS (not infection with the AIDS virus, or ARC) is currently a reportable disease in 45 states as well as the District of Columbia and Puerto Rico. In the future mandatory reporting of AIDS-related complex or merely infection with the AIDS virus may be required in many states.

94. Q. Should AIDS virus infection become a "reportable disease"?

A. Yes, but it raises the crucial question of how the rights of the infected people can be guaranteed. It is important to insure that making AIDS virus infection reportable to county and state health departments is a step in the direction of public health and not the oppression of a group with an already uncertain future.

There are, of course, advantages in making AIDS virus infection reportable. With data available on a large number of infected people, researchers can identify new risk groups, refine knowledge about transmission, and understand the role of cofactors leading to disease. However, maintaining confidentiality of the data is critically important to the success of these efforts.

Making AIDS virus infection a reportable disease without clear policies on the releasing of test results for insurance, employment, and prosecution (for violation of sodomy statutes) would court disaster. Individuals who suspect infection would avoid blood testing at all costs. This would neither help prevent the spread of the virus nor add to our understanding about the disease. It would likely drive underground those who suspect infection and create a class of angry, alienated people.

We are in the midst of an evolving national health emergency. Infected people have enough to worry about medically without having a series of financial and professional doors closing on them.

On September 18, 1985, the Colorado state board of public health ratified an earlier decision to make AIDS virus infection reportable. However well-intentioned this may have been, it will undoubtedly discourage those individuals who fear infection from having their blood tested. Widespread use of available alternate test-sites will be realized only when a positive outcome is made as "consequence-free" as possible. (See pages 230–233.)

95. **Q.** **Should children infected with the AIDS virus go to special schools?**

A. In some cases it would be wise to segregate infected children.

This fall there is a pattern of "AIDS hysteria" relating to infected children at school. Needless to say, this is an extremely emotional issue for parents. Because the AIDS virus cannot be transmitted by casual contact, AIDS-virus-positive students could attend school without putting classmates at risk as long as basic precautions are observed. In addition to the obvious (refraining from sexual contact and the sharing of needles), common-sense sanitation procedures should also be followed. Infected children should avoid contact sports and should not share food with other children.

The problem is deciding when a child has reached the age where he or she is responsible enough for his or her actions so that all kinds of exposure can be avoided. In younger children rough play, spitting, drooling, and biting all represent ways to transmit the virus.

Parents who wish to ban children with AIDS from schools should consider that there are a large number of infected, symptomless individuals. To be truly effective, a policy that bans children with ARC or AIDS should also include a provision to screen all students for AIDS virus infection. This would be dramatic and will probably only be considered in areas of high prevalence.

Parents and teachers should discourage rough, physical play. Teachers should be especially vigilant of this in younger children. Parents should also warn their children of the dangers of drugs. In some schools there is a serious drug problem, and the sharing of an infected needle puts an individual at risk for AIDS virus infection.

It should also be added that in the vast majority of situations children in school are not at risk for contracting the AIDS virus. There are no recorded examples of a child being infected by another in a school situation. Parents should also keep in mind that physicians who work with AIDS patients do not fear that proximity and do not believe that touching puts them or their loved ones at risk. Care should be taken so that parents do not consciously or unconsciously frighten their children unnecessarily about what is, in most situations, an extremely unlikely possibility.

96. Q. Could the AIDS virus be spread in an organized, evil way?

A. Yes. Certainly some infected, well-financed, promiscuous individuals could facilitate the spread of the AIDS virus into large segments of the population, nationally and globally, as part of a "dirty war." There is no evidence currently available to substantiate this wild but frightening supposition.

97. Q. What will AIDS cost society, and who will pay?

A. There are two prices that the AIDS virus will exact from our society. It will cost many lives and many dollars.

Dr. Ann Hardy, director of public health for the Centers for Disease Control, estimates that each AIDS case costs approximately three-quarters of a million dollars. There is $140,000 in direct outlay for medical expenses and approximately $600,000 lost to society in terms of future earnings of those who die.

There is no question that AIDS will put a phenomenal strain on our financial, emotional, and spiritual reserves. It can be predicted that by the end of the decade America will have more than 250,000 AIDS patients. That would mean more than $35 billion in direct outlays and *$150 billion* in lost future earnings.

The emotional loss cannot be measured in dry statistics. Terminal illness is always a tragic experience for family and loved ones. The fact that so many victims are in the prime of life adds to its impact. Unless the "tide is stemmed," the effect on our country of tens of thousands, hundreds of thousands, and perhaps millions of deaths due to AIDS is almost beyond comprehension.

98. Q. Has the AIDS virus spread from America to other parts of the world?

A. Yes. It is believed that the spread of the AIDS virus in Europe, North America, South America, Asia, and Australia was greatly facilitated by symptom-less carriers from the United States. Seven hundred seventy-eight cases of AIDS have been reported in the Americas from 14 countries other than the United States. The largest numbers have appeared in Haiti (340), Canada (190), and Brazil (182).[3] (See Figure 3–3.)

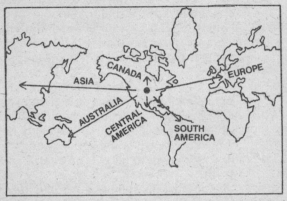

Figure 3-3. Spread of AIDS virus infection from the United States to the rest of the world.

99. Q. How big a problem is AIDS in Europe?

A. As of March 31, 1985, a total of 940 cases of European AIDS had been reported from France, Germany, England, Denmark, Switzerland, the Netherlands, Norway, Sweden, Finland, Spain, Italy, Austria, Greece, and Belgium to the World Health Organization, which is acting as a central collection agency for data. These cases had caused 468 deaths, for a fatality rate of 50%, which is quite similar to the American pattern.

AIDS has been recognized as a problem in France since 1981. By March 1985, 307 cases were reported. (See Figure 3–4.) French researchers were instrumental in isolating the AIDS virus. The French are also active in investigating a number of possible treatment programs for AIDS. Included in this is the controversial HPA-23, which has been approved by the FDA for limited clinical trials in the United States.

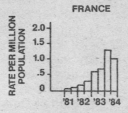

Figure 3-4. Incidence of acquired immune deficiency syndrome by 6-month period of diagnosis in France, through December 31, 1984.

Two countries with growing concern about the AIDS epidemic are England and Germany. (See Figure 3–5.) It seems that England is experiencing the same pattern of AIDS cases as America—with a four-year time lag. London and San Francisco also have similar patterns, once again with a four-year time difference.

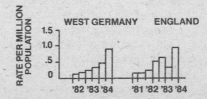

Figure 3-5. Incidence of acquired immune deficiency syndrome by 6-month period of diagnosis in Germany and England, through December 31, 1984.

Germans are extremely worried about the spread of the AIDS virus. Screening data suggests about 20% of all prostitutes are infected. Blood bank results from the first six months of testing were reported at the National Institutes of Health workshop on July 31, 1985. Germany reported that 0.24% of its donors were infected. This may be compared with the American estimate of 0.09%.

The recognition of the growing global AIDS epidemic is a challenge to the resourcefulness of the world's political leaders. AIDS calls for international cooperation and may be a topic on which the superpowers can work together.

100. Q. What recommendations has the World Health Organization (WHO) made in response to the AIDS epidemic?

   A. A number of members of the World Health Organization attended the International Conference on AIDS in Atlanta on April 15–17, 1985. WHO held its own meeting immediately thereafter and arrived at some recommendations to member nations:

   1) That member countries should inform the public about the methods of transmission of the AIDS virus so that individuals could take preventative measures.

   2) That member countries should make sure that its health care workers are trained to cope with AIDS patients' needs, including their psychosocial needs.

   3) That member countries should develop diagnostic procedures, including standardized blood tests.

   4) That blood-screening procedures should be implemented to protect the blood supply, with informed consent procedures in place.

   5) That organ, sperm, and tissue donations be screened for AIDS virus infection.

6) That individuals with a positive blood test for the AIDS virus should be referred for medical evaluation and counseling.

7) That laboratory procedures designed to protect health care workers from infection be developed and emphasized.

8) That blood samples from health care workers should be taken and stored on a regular basis to assess the risk of on-the-job infection.

9) That confidentiality for AIDS patients and AIDS-virus-positive individuals be respected.

CHAPTER 3 REFERENCES

1. CDC. Heterosexual transmission of human T-lymphotropic virus type III/lympadenopathy-associated virus, Morbid Mortal Weekly Rep 34:37, 1985.

2. DeJarlais D. *Heroin influx update.* New York, New York State, Division of Substance Abuse Services, Bureau of Research, 1983, review of public health services response to AIDS, p. 26.

3. Ginzburg H. HTLV inection in intravenous drug users, presented at HTLV Symposium, sponsored by the National Cancer Institute, National Institutes of Health, Bethesda, Maryland, December 6-7, 1984.

4. Salahuddin SZ, Markham PD, Popovic M, et al. Isolation of infectious human T-cell leukemia/lymphotropic virus type III (HTLV-III) from patients with acquired immunodeficiency syndrome (AIDS) or AIDS-related complex (ARC) and from healthy carriers: A study of risk groups and tissue sources. Proc Natl Acad Sci USA 82:5530, 1985.

5. Curran JW, Morgan WM, Hardy AM, et al. The epidemiology of AIDS: current status and future prospects. Science 229:1352, 1985.

6. Bross DC. Legal aspects of STD control. In *Sexually Transmitted Diseases.* Holmes KF, Mardh P, Sparling PF, Wiesnes PJ (eds). McGraw-Hill Book Company, New York, 1984, pp. 929-930.

4

Making Sex Safer

The basic methods by which the AIDS virus can be transmitted are well known—from contaminated blood, from sharing contaminated needles, from exchange of body fluids in sex, and from mother to infant or unborn child. Screening measures have virtually made the nation's blood supply safe from AIDS virus contamination. The problem of infected mothers transmitting the virus to their infant or unborn child is a growing but still relatively small problem. Warnings have been issued to those who use contaminated intravenous needles (in drug use) to avoid sharing needles. Clearly sexual transmission of the AIDS virus will remain the mode of transmission that threatens the greatest number of people.

What Is "Safe Sex" and Who Should Practice It?

Safe sex is sex in which precautions are taken to avoid an undesirable outcome. The term "safe sex" invites the query, "Safe from what?" Couples for centuries have taken a variety of measures to make sex "safer"—usually from the possibility of unwanted pregnancy or venereal disease. Couples attempting to utilize any method of birth control —rhythm, coitus interruptus, oral sex, masturbation, condoms, diaphragms, or the Pill, are all practicing a form of "safe sex." Someone who inspects a potential "first time" sexual partner for signs of herpes is also practicing a form of "safe sex." "Safe sex" has become a term widely used in homosexual communities to signify a set of safeguards specifically designed to avoid AIDS virus infection. This connotation will be implicit in this chapter and will undoubtedly become common with the growing recognition that AIDS threatens all sexually active people. Widespread public knowledge about safe sexual practices and, more important, their consistent implementation is the greatest hope for moderating the spread of the AIDS virus. Safe sex should be practiced by all sexually active individuals. Individuals who are married or presumably otherwise monogamously involved should also consider safe sex.

The AIDS virus arrived in this country by 1977, and that is the year often cited as the "cutoff" for possible infection. Current FDA guidelines recommend that any male who has had sex with another male since 1977, or whose sexual partner has had sex with another male since 1979, is asked to defer from donating blood due to the chance that they may be infected. This means that unless a couple has been in a *strictly* monogamous relationship for the past six years (heterosexual couple) or eight years (homosexual couple) the possibility that one or both may be a carrier of the AIDS virus should be considered.

A couple who has been married for 10 years hypothetically does not need to consider the topic of "safe sex." However, a number of surveys indicate that a large percentage of married people have had extramarital affairs. Husbands who have had contact with prostitutes (particularly in large cities) and wives who have had contact with bisexual men are certainly at risk for AIDS virus infection. Parents should, of course, be able to explain safe sex to their children and the reasons for it. Clearly, the topic of "safe sex" should be a personal concern for nearly all Americans.

What Is "Unsafe Sex" and Why Is It Unsafe?

Unsafe sexual practices are those that create a legitimate risk for transmission of the AIDS virus. Although it is self-evident, it is worth stating that it is impossible to become infected by a partner who is not a carrier. In other words, selection of a sexual partner has become one of the critical choices of the times in which we live. The choice of a "risky" sexual partner is perhaps the most unsafe sexual practice of all.

Promiscuity (multiple sexual partners) correlates more strongly than any specific sexual practice to AIDS virus infection. This holds true for both homosexuals and heterosexuals. It is clear that the "law of probabilities" holds true in this case—every new partner is also a new risk. Reducing the number of sexual partners is the sanest first step an individual can take toward eliminating unsafe sexual practices.

How is it possible to choose a "safe" partner? With 90% of the carriers of the AIDS virus symptomless, there is no way, short of a mutual blood test, for two partners to be absolutely sure that neither is infected. Trying to get a "general feel" for a prospective partner's sexual philosophy may be interesting but is of no consequence in determining whether or not they are actually infected. While the dictum "Know your partner" is a good guideline, it should not be used as a surrogate blood test. Good advice for today is to presume infection in a new partner until you know differently.

In addition to choice of partner there are 10 "rules of safe sex" (actually "rules for avoiding unsafe sex") which should be followed:

DURING SEX

1. Do not ingest semen.
2. Avoid oral contact with the vagina, rectum, or penis.

3. Do not receive ejaculated semen in the vagina, rectum, or mouth.
4. Do not injest urine.
5. Do not exchange saliva.
6. Do not have any kind of sex without washing with soap immediately afterward.
7. Do not have sex with multiple partners.

THINGS TO THINK ABOUT BEFORE SEX

8. Do not have sex if you have a fever.
9. Do not have sex when you know you are ill.
10. Do not indulge in immune-altering drugs (basically all recreational drugs and alcohol) when having sex.

How Can "Safe Sex" Be Enjoyable?

Individuals previously unfamiliar with the concept of "safe sex" (to avoid AIDS virus infection) are often shocked to read "the rules." A frequent response is, "It sounds too much like no sex." However, unless a definitely uninfected couple is enjoying a *completely* monogamous relationship, "safe sex" is an intelligent step in the direction of self-preservation.

There are a variety of practices that express love and affection without exposing the participants to infection. Sharing of orgasms, which is the "cement" of relationships and the *sine qua non* of recreational sex, is still quite possible. The only rule is, no exchange of body fluids. The quality of the sexual experience relies on love, creativity, and feedback. With conventional insertion of the penis into the vagina (or rectum) discouraged, individuals can adjust by finding sexual satisfaction in noncoital practices.

Couples facing abrupt changes in their sexual habits should be reassured by the admonition that there is no "normal" or "natural" way for sex to proceed. Sex researchers and counselors have maintained that "sex equals intercourse" is a misconception born out of popular myths and stereotypes. The assumption that intercourse ought to be the absolute conclusion to every sexual encounter has been called the "myth of coital primacy." Improvement of the sexual experience is accomplished by turning attention to overlooked but essential components, for example: touching, relaxation, masturbation training, communication, fantasies, and sharing of erotic needs.

Kissing, fondling, and manipulation of the genitals have been popularly regarded as subservient to sexual intercourse, as is implied in the word "foreplay." When the goal of sex is procreation, the indispensable component is intercourse. But when the goal of a sexual encounter is recreation, the emphasis on intercourse may distract many people from discovering practices they like very much and actually prefer. In their intelligent book, *Male Sexuality*, Bernie Zilbergeld and John Ullman cite one man who testified:

> For many years, while I enjoyed all kinds of sexual stimulation, I always insisted on "finishing" (coming) inside a vagina. I just "knew" that this was the best way. I was quite surprised when I finally allowed myself to climax with other types of stimulation. I enjoyed a sense of being done to or being taken care of that I rarely got with intercourse, and I found that I have the most explosive orgasms through hand stimulation. Of course, explosive orgasms and being taken care of are not the only things I want from sex, and intercourse is better at providing some of the other things I want. But now that I know what leads to what, I feel I have more options and can better choose one that will fit my wants at the moment![1]

In an age when many individuals will be substituting other means of stimulation for coitus, it is interesting to note that many will find they don't necessarily prefer to conclude their sexual experience by ejaculating inside the vagina (or, with male homosexuals, inside the rectum). They will be joined by men and women who don't ordinarily reach orgasm through intercourse but respond best to manual stimulation and will suffer not at all in the practice of safe sex. Some will regret the loss of oral sex as a coital substitute, only to realize this does not mean an end to sexual satisfaction. Oral sex, though pleasurable to many, is clearly not the only noncoital way to achieve orgasm and, depending on the couple, may not be the best or most enjoyable.

In safe sex, attention must be shifted from copulation to eroticizing nonrisk parts of the body. The techniques of this are largely unexplored, so each participant can become a sort of theoretician and pioneer in this important part of the times.

The adjustment to safe sex may be facilitated by the use of beautiful and simple sexual exercises that Masters and Johnson called "sensate focusing" but that sex therapist Helen Singer Kaplan prefers to call "pleasuring." The exercises begin with gentle caressing, stroking, and nuzzling all other parts of the body except the genitals. In many cases the feelings aroused are sensuous but not sexual, and enjoyment is gained through feelings for their own sake. The objective is to free the couple of sexual pressures and enhance the affectionate bond between people.

A subsequent exercise, genital pleasuring, involves stroking, fondling, and otherwise manually stimulating the genitals. The sensations are maintained without sexual intercourse and can be sustained without the pressure of sexual achievement. Again, the aim is used to build intimacy through the mutual enjoyment of pleasurable sensations.

Through these exercises couples can further eroticize nonrisk parts of the body through relaxation and focus. Individuals can therefore expand their personal universe of erogenous feelings and determine new kinds of stimulation they like.

Sexual communication training, useful in promoting mutual enjoyment in coitus, again has a place in safe sex. It involves exploring pleasurable stimulations and then communicating these effectively to one's sexual partner. Couples are encouraged to make greater use of imagery and imagination, encouraging fantasies which are playful and sexually safe.

It is a well-known fact that most humans fantasize during sex. It is the internal component of the sexual act, patterned by learning and imagination, unique from person to person. The images and reveries of erotic fantasy are possibly more important in safe sex than in sex in general. Fantasies are especially valuable when shared between partners, which helps build trust and intimacy. They are a practice, particularly when acted upon, which can often be done within the guidelines of safe sex.

Interestingly, the focus of most sexual fantasies is not sexual acts at all. Rather, they more often focus on imaginary roles, partners, places, and situations. Their function is to intensify the sexual experience.

When "unsafe" sexual practices (oral sex, etc.) are central to the fantasy, it is always possible to preserve safe sex by retaining the mental images but changing the sex act itself.

The following is a partial listing of love techniques that present an acceptable degree of risk.

"SAFE" SEXUAL PRACTICES

TOUCHING

BREASTS: palm brushing, eyelid brushing, sucking, licking.

BUTTOCKS: holding, kneading, slapping, beating.

PENIS: stroking, tickling, oil massage.

VAGINA: gentle fingering, manually stimulating clitoris and vulva.

EARS: gentle fingering of the auricle and earlobe.

WHOLE BODY: relaxation massage, oil massage.

FEET: tickling, erogenic stimulation through pressing various zones such as the instep.

GENITALIA: mutual handwork in all couples, caressing pubic hair.

KISSING
Breasts and nipples, shoulders, neck, armpits, fingers, palms, toes, soles of feet, navel, scrotum, ears and earlobes.

SUCKING
Breasts, earlobes, fingers, toes.

MASTURBATION
Mutual masturbation, observing each other masturbating, masturbation as a learning tool in sensory awareness, mutual handwork, group stimulation.

PENETRATION SURROGATES
Femoral intercourse (inserting the penis into the space between the thighs, below the crotch), intermammary intercourse (inserting the penis between the breasts), rubbing the penis against the belly; all usually performed with oil lubrication.

STIMULATION THROUGH FRICTION
Mutual genital friction, vaginal stimulation with thigh, stimulating the penis in the fold of the elbow, the fold of the knee, or the hair.

Is There a Less Restrictive Form of "Safe Sex"?

Yes, though it must be remembered that projections of "relative risk" are speculative and hypothetical. An individual who becomes infected through *any* sexual contact would find little consolation in learning that the activity which led to it was "relatively safe." Once again, it is "safe" for two uninfected people to have sex. It is "unsafe" for an uninfected person to have sex with a carrier. The optimal model (from the point of view of "safety") for an uninfected individual is to develop a completely monogamous relationship with another uninfected individual.

It is possible to make informed speculation, however, about practices that may not be completely "safe" but represent less of a risk than "unsafe" practices. A truly paranoid individual, obsessed with a fear of infection with the AIDS virus, could no doubt find cause for suspicion in any contact with other humans, sexual or not. Entrepreneurial attempts to exploit the fear of AIDS by marketing such devices as "AIDS Public Telephone Mouthpiece Protectors" (a custom-made piece of disposable wax paper) testify to this. While the AIDS epidemic will no doubt cause a surfacing of fringe individuals with a "Howard Hughes complex," a majority will hopefully opt for a more rational approach. The elimination of the greatest risk factors, most notably unsafe sexual practices, will go a long way to preventing infection and maintaining emotional equilibrium.

Obviously there is a "hierarchy of relative risk." An individual driven by self-destructive (or even suicidal) impulses, could hypothetically risk life-threatening infection by consciously and blatantly "breaking all the rules" of safe sex. He or she might, for example, try to develop a flu, ingest immune-suppressing drugs, seek out a man known to be infected, and practice receptive anal intercourse without the benefit of lubricant. The other extreme of the continuum would be the person who swears to a life of celibacy in order to avoid AIDS. Between these end points there are a variety of activities that represent different degrees of risk.

In trying to assess "relative risk," it is important to remember that there are three critical variables in transmission—mode of transmission, dose of contagion, and condition of host at the time of exposure.

Mode of transmission—How does the (possibly infectious) body fluid become exposed? Anal, vaginal, and oral sex are risky because sensitive mucosal membranes are exposed. Mutual masturbation is less risky because it would likely require a cut or abrasion of the skin to create a portal to the bloodstream.

Dose of contagion—How much virus is contained in the transmitted body fluid? Infected semen has an extremely high concentration of virus; saliva less so. Thus "French" kissing, while not completely "safe," is less risky than oral sex (in which there is contact with semen, delicate areas of the penis, or vaginal secretions).

Condition of host at time of exposure—An individual who is sick or has an otherwise damaged immune system is apparently at greater risk for contracting the AIDS virus. Thus you should avoid sex if you are feeling generally ill, especially "feverish."

Other speculations into "less safe" sex include the use of contraceptive devices. Condoms have been used to prevent the spread of sexually transmitted disease and should reduce the risk of the AIDS virus infection. However, condoms rupture (some say 20% of the time), in which case they lose their effectiveness. There are indications that nonoxynol-9, frequently found in spermicidal jelly, will kill the AIDS virus. Thus it is probable that its use as a lubricant (in combination with a condom) in penile-rectal sex and with a condom and diaphragm in penile-vaginal sex may reduce risk. Another "less safe" approach is the use of a condom in oral-penile sex. In using lubricants with condoms, care must be taken *not* to use oil-based products such as Vaseline (which can emulsify and weaken latex condoms). K-Y jelly is recommended.

French kissing can be classified as a "less safe" form of sex as well. Though one case of AIDS virus transmission as an apparent result of intimate kissing has been recorded, this is presumed to be a lower risk activity due to a lower dose of contagion in saliva and the (unproven) supposition that gastric acid of the stomach may kill the AIDS virus.

Important Note—Careful washing with soap is an important component of "safe sex," in order to remove residues of secretions which may contain infectious material.

How Can I Overcome My Reluctance to Start Practicing Safe Sex?

OBJECTION #1
"I am afraid to ask my partner to practice safe sex with

me."—The times we live in have presented us with a new etiquette born of necessity. It is now acceptable to inform your partner that you practice safe sex. In fact, it is now OK to demand it. A person who says no has probably said no before and is therefore practicing *unsafe* sex. That person is a bad risk to begin with.

OBJECTION #2

"Chances are we're infected already, so why bother?"— Don't start with this defeatist view. You don't *know* if you're infected without a blood test. If you are AIDS virus positive, you have a responsibility to your sexual partners. A more constructive attitude is to consider yourself *not* infected unless you know differently. Safe sex can be an affirmative choice you make for your own well-being.

OBJECTION #3

"I can't stop kissing, so I might as well go all the way."— Kissing and the exchange of semen are not comparable, risk-wise. If it is impossible for you to give up kissing, why not stop the risk there? A kiss is no reason to divest yourself of all safeguards and engage in higher risk sexual activities.

OBJECTION #4

"I don't want to be locked into safe sex forever."—When you begin a new relationship, it is prudent to conduct safe sex until you and your partner have developed enough commitment to want to take the AIDS virus blood test together. If both partners are negative, the couple can feel more confident in expanding their sexual practices.

In the event that one of the partners tests positive, the couple should continue safe sex indefinitely. Religious or personal counseling may also provide guidance to couples whose relationship is strained by this unpleasant news.

If *both* partners test positive, safe sex should still be

continued. The fact that both are infected with the AIDS virus does not mean they have nothing to lose. A positive blood test does not necessarily mean you will develop the disease.

Furthermore, the partners run the risk of transmitting *other* viruses to each other, and the multiple-variants theory (see question 81) postulates that infection by more than one variant of the AIDS virus may be an important cofactor in an individual's development of ARC or the full-blown syndrome. There is no wisdom in taking the risk that your loved one's contagion may "tip the balance."

OBJECTION #5
"Safe sex is not satisfying."—This is emphatically untrue. Any orgasm is sexually satisfying. Intimacy and closeness do not require the exchange of bodily fluids, and there are alternatives. What you can do without risk may be more pleasurable than you think. If there *is* any loss of pleasure, it is not a complete loss. The price you pay may be well worth it in terms of your peace of mind and the amount of risk you avoid.

Does "Safe Sex" Represent a Real Hope?

The promiscuity that led in great part to the spread of the AIDS epidemic seems to be abating, calling into question the value of the modern sexual revolution. Popular focus in the 1980s seems to be switching from sexual freedom and mobility to commitment and monogamous lifestyles. People are more prepared, temperamentally, for the long haul, and even eager for the security of lasting relationships. But are they prepared for the discipline of safe sex?

The recent statistics on the decline of sexually transmitted diseases, which has been attributed to a change in sexual practices by male homosexuals in response to the AIDS threat, is encouraging. The numbers indicate the homosexual population is effectively revising its sexual habits in response to the threat of a disease. This phenomenon is historic insofar as it displays the impact of information campaigns and an unprecedented willingness on the part of individuals to take responsibility for sexual behavior.

Perhaps it represents a positive result of the now much maligned sexual revolution; perhaps it is just a reaction to the severity of the AIDS threat. Whether it indicates that modern Americans are growing up or just acquiring a discipline born of necessity, it is a hopeful sign. The question then becomes, can we keep it up? Will heterosexuals follow the gay example? For now, safe sex seems a workable plan and a practical response to the spread of AIDS and our own feelings of helplessness in these troubled times.

Allen M. Brandt wrote in the conclusion to his landmark social history of venereal disease in America, *No Magic Bullet*:

> If anything has become clear in the course of the twentieth century it is that behavior is subject to complex forces, internal psychologies and external pressures, all not subject to immediate modification, or, arguably, to modification at all. Sexuality is subject to a number of powerful influences, social and economic, conscious and unconscious, many more powerful than are suggested by the prescriptive sexual education that some advocate, many more powerful than even the fear of venereal disease. In this view, sexuality is equated with other risk-taking behavior—smoking, drinking, poor diet, driving too fast. These are behaviors for which, of course, individuals can in part be held accountable, but the question of to what extent, and whether they should be is not as simple.[2]

Brandt concludes that the American way to control venereal disease is to stress individual responsibility, but concedes that it has failed to control VD so far. The flaw in such efforts, he asserts persuasively, is our tendency to view VD as a punishment for sexual misbehavior and an index of social decay.

In this context, safe sex as a voluntary revision of sexual habits may succeed if it can be adopted free of the stigma of social guilt. Considering the universally fatal nature of the disease, "safe sex" must become for us a discipline born of necessity, not a punishment for previous sin. "Safe sex" challenges us with adopting a more enlightened and sensitive view of sexual pleasure and goals. The pressures of a feared epidemic may well inspire us to adapt our relationships to a higher sensitivity, with attendant benefits to our own growth and to the community at large.

Why Was This Chapter Included in This Book?

The authors did not begin this project with the idea in mind of writing a book, or even a chapter, on sexual practices. As the book was being written, we realized that it would be incomplete, in fact irresponsible, to ignore this subject or treat it with clinical detachment. Some will be offended by what they consider as excessive graphic detail. Others will no doubt feel that this has been a cursory or shallow treatment of *the* most important topic about the AIDS epidemic.

To those who wish for a more in-depth treatment of the subject, we would like to suggest that a number of "how to" sex books are available. Although they may not be written with a "safe sex" slant, by applying knowledge of how to reduce the risk of transmission, they can be easily adapted as such.

To those who are shocked and offended, we would like to empathize with your immediate reaction. This is not a topic that is easy to discuss, but our nation is being confronted with a strange and frightening disease that knows no rules nor recognizes any proprieties. As unpleasant as these topics may be, none of us is exempt from the responsibility of informing those we love about what can be done to combat AIDS.

We have recently observed a national mobilization against drunk driving. Television, radio, and magazine advertisements remind us that "friends don't let friends drive drunk." By the end of this decade, more people may be dying of AIDS than are killed in auto accidents. We each have a moral obligation to see to it that no one is without the information that may protect him or her from this deadly disease.

CHAPTER 4 REFERENCES

1. Zilbergeld B, Ullman J. *Male Sexuality: A guide to Sexual Fulfillment*, Little, Brown and Company, Boston, p. 51, 1978.
2. Brandt AM. *No Magic Bullet, A Social History of Venereal Diseases in the United States Since 1880*, Oxford University Press, New York, p. 186, 1985.

II

THE AIDS EPIDEMIC: PAST, PRESENT AND FUTURE

5

Beginnings of a Global Epidemic

The AIDS virus, or one of its ancestors, infected humans in small numbers in central Africa in the early 1970s. Information from Africa is scarce due in part to a lack of medical care. The AIDS virus could have caused deaths in the early 1970s, or possibly the virus that first infected humans evolved into a more virulent form first, causing African AIDS cases in the late 1970s.

A study of 75 samples of blood saved from use in other studies in Uganda showed that 50 (67%) contained antibodies for the AIDS virus.[1] These samples were collected between August 1972 and July 1973, from a group of children with a mean age of 6.4 years.

The fact that these children were healthy at the time of the study is interesting. (They comprised a control group for a study of an endemic lymphoma.) One possibility is that the children had some sort of natural immunity to the AIDS virus. A second possibility is that many of these children will go on to develop longer range complications.

A third possibility is that the strain of AIDS virus in their blood was a predecessor to a more virulent strain. There have been at least 18 different variations of the AIDS virus isolated to date and it is possible that some are more powerful than others.[2] In any case, this study is the earliest indication of AIDS virus found in humans anywhere in the world.[1]

The AIDS virus apparently made its way into humans from African green monkeys, or *Cercopithecus aethiops.* Dr. Max Essex of the Harvard School of Public Health has studied this connection.[3] He found that 42% of a group of healthy green monkeys had blood that indicated AIDS virus infection. He found no such evidence in groups of baboons and chimpanzees. Green monkeys are unique among African lower primates in that they are proximate and interactive with human populations. Other viruses have made the leap from animals to humans in the past, including yellow fever virus.[4] Investigators speculate the AIDS virus was first transmitted from green monkeys to man by bites, bestial sex, or slaughter for food and clothing. A detailed structural analysis of the AIDS virus by Dr. Robert Gallo at the National Cancer Institute (NCI) supports Dr. Essex' contention. The variants recovered from Zairian AIDS patients are the human variants that most closely resemble the virus found in green monkeys.

The AIDS virus made its way to the Western hemisphere from Africa in the 1970s. After AIDS was defined by the Centers for Disease Control in 1981, a search of medical records revealed that the first known case of AIDS in the Western Hemisphere appears to have taken place in Haiti. A previously healthy 20-year-old man was diagnosed in July 1978 with biopsy-proven toxoplasmosis of the central nervous system. It is now believed that he was suffering from AIDS.[5]

Haiti does not have the kind of centralized reporting procedures that exist in America. Nevertheless, from available evidence, it appears that AIDS cases began cropping up rapidly in Haiti in 1980. Haitian AIDS resembles

American AIDS in that it centers around cities. However, 30% of the reported Haitian AIDS cases are female, which is three times the proportion in America. One third of Haitian men who have AIDS are either bisexual or have served as homosexual prostitutes for tourists.[5]

It is now believed that a period of two years or more elapses between infection with the virus and the development of AIDS. Therefore it is possible to make some inferences about the early spread of the virus in Haiti. The AIDS virus appears to have entered the Haitian population in 1976 or 1977 and grown rapidly beginning in 1978. (The small number of reports that seemed to indicate AIDS in 1978–1979 and the increase in 1980 would bear this out.)

Testing of blood samples indicates AIDS virus infection occurred in America by 1977 and spread geographically by 1980. There were 13 cases of Kaposi's sarcoma, *Pneumocystis carinii*, or perianal herpes in homosexual men recorded in 1978–1979.[6] While these reports were being classified in 1981 as the first American cases of AIDS,[7] the infection rate of the virus was taking a profound leap.

The similarities in timing and growth of the Haitian and American spread of AIDS suggest that the virus was introduced into the two populations at about the same time. It is possible that vacationing American gay men were infected with the virus and brought it back to the United States, since Haiti is a favorite vacation spot for affluent Americans and many Haitian men with a history of acting as homosexual prostitutes for tourists have developed the disease. It is also possible that Haitian immigrants brought the virus with them to American cities.

The appearance of AIDS in both Haiti and America several years after the virus appeared in humans in Africa raises the question of how it made its journey from Africa to the West. There are two theories about this. Dr. Peter Piot of the Institute of Tropical Medicine in Belgium has observed that several thousand Haitians lived in Kinshasa, Zaire, from the early 1960s to the mid-1970s and many of them have since moved to North America and Europe, perhaps carrying the AIDS virus with them.[8]

A second theory is that Cuban soldiers fighting in Angola may have acquired the virus and brought it back to the West with them. The proximity of Cuba to Haiti and the fact that Haitian AIDS is related to urban prostitution is suggestive. The AIDS virus is quite prevalent in central Africa. It is possible that Cuban mercenaries originally picked up the virus in Africa and brought it to Haiti, infecting urban prostitutes. There is anecdotal evidence that there were a number of Cuban soldiers in northern Angola in 1977.[9] This places them close to Zaire, which now has 8–12% of its adult population infected with the AIDS virus.[10-13]

As Dr. Jacques Leibowitch reported, "In 1977–78, the Cuban government expelled a certain number of undesirables among whom figured magalitas [homosexuals] and Angola veterans. A certain number of the latter found refuge in Florida, in Miami. Miami and southeast Florida is [sic] a recognized zone of 'swinging' homosexual activity, a boat-trip from the island of heterosexual protectionism. Miami, a $95 round trip from Port-Au-Prince, exotic turntable of the American and Caribbean worlds. Miami, linked to them by long chains of homosexual fraternity of the type Miami-Haiti, Los Angeles-Haiti, New York-Haiti-Miami. Thus might have been born a new epidemic, out of the jungle depths of Africa, into the Western world."[9]

Once the AIDS virus made its "beachhead" in America it spread through urban male homosexuals to other groups. Urban male homosexuals made up more than 80% of the first 300 AIDS cases.[14] The virus soon spread to another group—intravenous drug users. The virus can be transmitted very efficiently from the sharing of contaminated needles, and 8% of the homosexual men who develop AIDS also use intravenous drugs.[6] Thus the virus achieved a "portal of entry" into a new population. The first case of AIDS in an intravenous drug user who was not a male homosexual appeared in 1980, and there was an explosive increase in this category in 1981.[6] We can therefore suppose that infection was spreading among intravenous drug users during 1979.

The practice of sharing contaminated intravenous needles gave the AIDS virus an opening to another group—urban prostitutes. Intravenous drug use is common among prostitutes, particularly those of the "streetwalking" class. Some prostitutes support the drug habits of their regular lovers in addition to their own. Thus the AIDS virus had access to another population segment outside the core group of those originally infected.

One more population infected with the AIDS virus prior to 1981 was hemophiliacs.[15] Hemophiliacs are routinely exposed to as many as a million blood samples a year through the use of Factor VIII, a blood-clotting agent made up of blood from literally thousands of donors. The practice among intravenous drug users of selling blood with which to buy drugs is a plausible explanation of the contamination of the blood supply. During 1981, the cause of AIDS remained a mystery to medical investigators. By the time that AIDS was first *defined*, the virus was already active in a number of different populations.

The first clue that "something was amiss" in America appeared in May 1981. Five cases of *Pneumocystis carinii* were reported in previously healthy homosexual men in Los Angeles. *Pneumocystis* is an extremely rare lung infection. It was previously seen mostly in transplant or chemotherapy patients taking certain types of drugs.

Because of the unusual pattern of this outbreak, a report was filed with the Centers for Disease Control (CDC) in Atlanta. The CDC is a federal agency that is responsible for keeping track of trends that may affect the public health. Each week the CDC publishes the *Morbidity and Mortality Weekly Report (MMWR)*, a categorical analysis of recent deaths and diseases.

The *MMWR* of June 5, 1981, reported and analyzed the five cases of *Pneumocystis carinii.*[16] It noted that *Pneumocystis* occurred almost exclusively in patients whose immune systems were severely suppressed. It was noted in the *MMWR* that all five patients, two of whom had died by the time of the report, had used inhalant drugs such as amyl nitrite or isobutyl nitrite. The five men, all previously healthy, were sexually active homosexuals between the ages of 29 and 36. Simultaneously, a number of cases of Kaposi's sarcoma appeared in homosexual men in San Francisco and New York City. These previously healthy men also showed evidence of immune dysfunction.

In the July 3, 1981, *MMWR* this unexpected outbreak of unusual illness was analyzed.[17] By this point, 26 cases of Kaposi's sarcoma and an additional 10 cases of *Pneumocystis carinii* had been recorded. All of the patients were from New York or California. The *MMWR* also noted that 4 homosexual men from New York City had been diagnosed as having severe suppression of the immune system in conjunction with herpes simplex infection. Three of these patients had died.

This pattern of rare, deadly disease accompanying a severely damaged immune system caused alarm at the Centers for Disease Control, which held a meeting in June 1981 to discuss the subject. The discussion group, headed by Dr. James Curran, decided that more information was needed. In order to expedite the collection of that information, they had to name and define the disease. They called it the "acquired immune deficiency syndrome," which became shortened to the acronym AIDS.

AIDS was defined as the presence of either *Pneumocystis carinii* or Kaposi's sarcoma in an otherwise healthy individual. "Acquired" was used because it was evident that it was not inherited. "Immune deficiency" described the link between Kaposi's sarcoma and *Pneumocystis carinii*. It was called a "syndrome" because the different manifestations were signs of one disease.

The Centers for Disease Control asked physicians around the country to report any cases of AIDS. With the standardized definition, it was hoped that information could be gathered and analyzed and some light shed on what was going on.

During the summer of 1981, AIDS cases started appearing rapidly, not only in the United States but also in Europe. Nearly 100 AIDS cases appeared in the United States during the summer of 1981. They were uniformly found in homosexual men in New York and California.

Early theories about AIDS attempted to link it to the lifestyle of the male, urban, gay community. Some of the speculation was wild. For example, one of the theories was that the breakdown of the immune system had something to do with excessive ultraviolet exposure from urban tanning salons. Another theory postulated drugs: it was thought that a bad batch of "poppers" (amyl nitrite or isobutyl nitrite), used as a sexual stimulant by homosexual men, would be discovered. Another group believed that AIDS could be due to a weakening of the immune system by exposure to multiple partners' semen. Other investigators suggested that sexually transmitted diseases, common in homosexual men, set the stage for AIDS by "burning out" the immune system.

It became obvious that, whatever its cause, AIDS was deadly. Patients who had it usually died within 18 months of diagnosis. AIDS patients were victimized by severe weight loss, persistent fever and diarrhea, night sweats, dry cough, mental deterioration, and coma. Because it was not understood how AIDS was transmitted, many of the victims were ostracized by family, friends, and even the medical community.

Throughout gay America, and particularly in large cities, the word began to spread. AIDS was frightening because it was deadly and so much was unknown. It became known as the "gay plague." A feeling of helplessness pervaded many gay communities. Stories began to circulate of young men, in the prime of life, falling victim to this undefined enemy. Information spread about what to look for. As 1981 drew to a close, more than 250 cases of AIDS had been diagnosed in the United States, while confusion persisted in the medical community.

During 1982 the Centers for Disease Control continued to work intently trying to determine the cause of AIDS. A significant step in the evolution of the CDC study was taken when three new groups unexpectedly emerged as being at risk for the development of AIDS—hemophiliacs, intravenous drug users, and recent Haitian immigrants. Although the new facts were confusing to investigators at the time, we now realize that these new types of cases were due to the spread of the virus in 1979–1981, before AIDS had been defined.

The Centers for Disease Control was particularly interested in the outbreak of AIDS among hemophiliacs.[16-17] This strongly suggested that the syndrome could be transmitted through the blood supply, and implied that the nation's blood banks might be contaminated. Blood banks went to work, discouraging blood donations by individuals from these groups who were now believed to be at high risk for AIDS. The findings in recent Haitian immigrants were something that caused both confusion and consternation among medical investigators. This information didn't seem to "fit" with any other factors known to be associated with AIDS. It was initially suggested that Haitians might possess some sort of inherent susceptibility to AIDS.

A later, more intensive analysis yielded the information that Haitian immigrants who came to America after 1978 were 40 times more likely to have AIDS than those who had immigrated prior to 1978.[10] It was eventually concluded that the prevalence of AIDS in Haitian immigrants was due to exposure to its causative agent, and not some sort of genetic deficiency. But this conclusion was not reached until 1984. As the evidence unfolded in 1982, the presence of AIDS in Haitians was another in a series of puzzling facts about this growing, deadly disease.

The emergence of hemophiliacs, intravenous drug users, and Haitian immigrants as risk groups destroyed the theory that AIDS was a "gay" disease. Investigators were directed to look for an infectious germ that could be transmitted through the blood and perhaps by other means. Epidemiologists continued the tedious process of comparative analysis—hoping to find a common thread that would help "break" the case.

A completely different "angle of attack" was provided by cell biologists. Dr. Robert Gallo of the National Cancer Institute began to investigate the possibility that AIDS was caused by a very specific type of germ, known as a retrovirus. Dr. Gallo had discovered the first human cancer virus in 1978, human T-cell leukemia virus (HTLV-I). This virus attacks the immune system and causes a rare and potent form of cancer. By the summer of 1982, Dr. Gallo had concluded that AIDS might also be caused by a human retrovirus, one that was previously unknown. HTLV-I was known to attack T-cells. Dr. Gallo observed that AIDS also attacked a type of T-cells and rendered them unable to perform their vital function. This reinforced his belief that AIDS was caused by a retrovirus.

This line of thought was supported by work done by Dr. Max Essex. Dr. Essex had been among the first to identify a virus, specifically a retrovirus, as the cause of leukemia in cats. When this virus attacked cats, some developed T-cell leukemia. In other cats a pattern quite similar to AIDS was produced—immune deficiency leaving the animal open to opportunistic infection.[20,21] These similarities further encouraged Dr. Gallo to search for a retrovirus as the cause of AIDS.

As 1982 drew to a close, it was becoming clear that AIDS was a deadly, infectious disease. More and more people were being diagnosed with AIDS each month. The outbreak of AIDS beyond the male homosexual community made it obvious that AIDS was not just a "gay disease." The question that loomed large as 1983 began was: "*If AIDS is not a gay disease, what is it?*"

CHAPTER 5 REFERENCES

1. Saxinger WC, Levine PH, Dean AG, et al. Evidence for exposure to HTLV-III in Uganda before 1973. Science 227:1036, 1985.
2. Wong-Staal F, Shaw GM, Hahn BH, et al. Genomic diversity of human T-lymphotropic virus type III (HTLV-III). Science 229:759, 1985.
3. Kanki PJ, Kurth R, Becker W, et al. Antibodies to simian T-lymphotropic retrovirus type III in African green monkeys and recognition of STLV-III viral proteins by AIDS and related sera. Lancet 1:1330, 1985.
4. Monath TP. Glad tidings from yellow fever research. Science 229:734, 1985.
5. Goedert JJ, Blattner WA. The epidemiology of AIDS and related conditions. *In AIDS: Etiology, Diagnosis, Treatment, and Preventions.* DeVita VT, Hellman S, Rosenberg SA (eds). J.B. Lippencott Company, New York, p. 1-30, 1985.
6. Hardy AM, Allen JR, Morgan WM. The incidence rate of acquired immunodeficiency syndrome in selected populations. JAMA 253:215, 1985.
7. CDC Task Force on Kaposi's Sarcoma and Opportunistic Infections: Epidemiologic aspects of the current outbreak of Kaposi's sarcoma and opportunistic infection. N Engl J Med 306:248, 1982.
8. Piot P, Taelman H, Minlanger KB, et al. Acquired immunodeficiency syndrome in a heterosexual population in Zaire. Lancet 2:65, 1984.
9. Leibowitch J (trans Howard R). *A Strange Virus of Unknown Origin.* Ballantine Books, New York, p. 68-9, 1985.
10. Quinn TC, Piot P, McCormick J, et al. Serologic and immunologic studies on HTLV-III and other infections in African and U.S. AIDS patients (abst). International Conference on Acquired Immunodeficiency Syndrome (AIDS), Atlanta, GA, April 14-17, 1985, p. 84.

11. Biggar RJ, Johnson B, Gigase P, et al. Seroepidemiology of HTLV-III in Eastern Zaire and Kenya (abst), International Conference on Acquired Immunodeficiency Syndrome (AIDS), Atlanta, GA, 1985, p. 68.

12. Biggar RJ. Melbye M, Kestems L, et al. Kaposi's sarcoma in Zaire is not associated with HTLV-III infection (letter). N Engl J Med 311:1051, 1984.

13. Brun-Vezinet F, Rouzioux C, Montagnier L, et al. Prevalence of antibodies to lymphadenopathy associated retrovirus in African patients with AIDS. Science 226:453, 1984.

14. Selik RM, Haverkos HW, Curran JW. Acquired immunodeficiency syndrome (AIDS) trends in the United States, 1978-82. Am J Med 76:493, 1984.

15. Evatt BL, Gomperts ED, McDougal JS. Coincidental appearance of LAV/HTLV-III antibodies in hemophiliacs and the onset of the AIDS epidemic. N Engl J Med 312:483, 1985.

16. Pneumocystis carinii pneumonia among patients with hemophilia A. Morbid Mortal Weekly Rep 31:365, 1982.

17. Update on acquired immunodeficiency syndrome (AIDS) among patients with hemophilia A. Morbid Mortal Weekly Rep 31:644, 1982.

18. Pape JW, Liautaud B, Thomas F, et al. Characteristics of the acquired immunodeficiency syndrome (AIDS) in Haiti. N Engl J Med 309:945, 1983.

19. Malebranche R, Arnoux E, Guerin JM, et al. Acquired immunodeficiency syndrome with severe gastrointestinal manifestations in Haiti. Lancet 2:873, 1983.

20. Trainin Z, Essex M. Immune response to tumor cells in domestic animals. J Am Vet Med Assoc 181:1125, 1982.

21. Hardy Jr, WD. Feline leukemia virus non-neoplastic diseases. J Am Animal Hosp Assoc 17:941, 1981.

6

Killer Exposed

As 1983 began, the rate at which AIDS cases were being diagnosed was increasing rapidly, and there was no apparent "leveling off" in sight. Due to the spread of AIDS outside the homosexual community, national press attention increased dramatically. Gay activists clamored for more government funding. Others used the outbreak as an excuse to violate the civil liberties of those in the identifiable high-risk groups. Gays were thrown off buses in San Francisco and Haitian immigrants were asked to move out of their apartments in New York. This public attention put a great deal of pressure on the ones who were expected to supply some sort of answer. Medical investigators, accustomed to working in an isolated, detached environment, felt the heat of public interest. Physicians who were on the "front line" treating AIDS patients felt a sense of helplessness and frustration as they witnessed disfigurement and death in hundreds of young people.

Dr. James Curran described his first direct encounter with AIDS:

I remember the first patient that I met. He was a highly educated, very intelligent, and extremely pleasant and open gay man. He had skin lesions of Kaposi's sarcoma. He took his clothes off, walked around the room, showed himself to all the doctors, and said, "Doctor, do you think this is serious? And you from the Centers for Disease Control, who've never seen a case of this before, what do you think?" And I acted like a doctor, and said, "Well, we hope not." As if I knew.

It was through continued collaboration with NYU that I was able to see this man on several more occasions before he died—only to develop progressive cancer, lose progressive weight, lose all his hair from chemotherapy, develop *Pneumocystis* pneumonia, brain infections, and finally die, a miserable death several months later.

And I think back on the time when I first saw the patient, and talked to him. He was from my home state. Talked to him about his days at an Ivy League school. What it was like to be gay in Detroit, if you will.... And we were talking about my, my, I'm a medical oddity, and you're a doctor who studies medical oddities, what do we think of each other. Only to realize that it wasn't fair. I'm still studying it and he's dead.*

The *Morbidity and Mortality Weekly Report* of March 4, 1983, attempted to summarize what was known about transmission pattern.[1] For the first time heterosexual spread was identified as a threat. A number of AIDS cases had appeared in female partners of men who were either AIDS patients or members of high-risk groups for AIDS.[2,3] AIDS was also reported to have been transmitted from mother to child.[4,5] The risk factor of Haitian immigrants was still a puzzling matter.[6-8]

The idea that immune suppression was widespread in certain high-risk populations was also documented. One study of New York homosexual men showed a large number having some degree of immune suppression.[9] This was

* Nova #1205. AIDS Chapter One. WGBH Transcripts (PBS), Broadcast on February 12. 1985.

also noted in a study with hemophiliacs.[10] These findings indicated that the same agent that caused AIDS evidently affected a much, much larger number of people. It also showed that individuals reacted differently to the presence of the agent—namely it was not always fatal within the first few years of infection. This news was comforting in that it suggested that not all infected individuals were doomed. But it raised the possibility that infection with the agent that caused AIDS was likely much more widespread than originally believed.

The March 4, 1983, *MMWR* went on to alert physicians to the following groups, believed to be at high risk for developing AIDS: those with signs or symptoms suggestive of AIDS, sexual partners of AIDS patients, sexually active homosexuals or bisexual men with multiple partners, present or past users of intravenous drugs, patients with hemophilia, and sexual partners of individuals at risk for AIDS. This definition "widened the net" considerably. The customer of a prostitute who was also an intravenous drug user was identified as being at risk, as were partners of sexually active bisexual men. Thus the shadow of doubt began to cast itself into the heterosexual world.

A number of agencies began disseminating information to try and educate the public, particularly those believed to be at high risk. Statements on prevention and control of AIDS were made by the American Association of Blood Banks, the American Association of Physicians for Human Rights, the American Red Cross, the Council of Community Blood Centers, the National Gay Task Force, and the National Hemophilia Foundation. Epidemiologists at the CDC continued to analyze carefully the commonalities among AIDS patients, hoping for the critical insight that would help identify the cause.

Meanwhile, in the United States Dr. Robert Gallo spearheaded the research effort at the National Cancer Institute. In France the two primary contributors were Dr. Willy Rosenbaum of the French Working Group and Dr. Luc Montagnier of the Pasteur Institute. These two groups ran nearly parallel paths. Both groups focused on the site of the attack—the T-helper cells of the body's immune system.

AIDS had a number of characteristic clinical manifestations. One critical indication was a reverse in an important ratio between two types of white blood cells: These are "T-helper" and "T-suppressor" cells. T-helper cells (described in Chapter 2) help to "rally the troops" in case of an invasion of hostile germs. T-suppressor cells perform a function that reverses the command of the T-helper cells. When an infection has been destroyed, the T-suppressor cells send out the message to "call off the troops." Together they make up the command structure of the immune system.

In the blood of normal, healthy individuals, there are *twice as many T-helper cells as T-suppressor cells.* In AIDS patients this ratio is reversed: there are twice as many T-suppressor cells as T-helper cells. We now realize that this is because the AIDS virus kills T-helper cells. More accurately stated, AIDS patients suffer from a lack of T-helper cells. In 1983 this mechanism was not understood. But the reversal in ratio provided a direction for research efforts.

In France and America research scientists attempted to isolate and study T-cells from AIDS patients. Dr. Gallo went through two frustrating sets of experiments in which he failed to culture the virus from isolated T-cells. The National Cancer Institute is well known for the ability to culture cells in similar experiments. But, for some reason, the T-cells did not grow in either experiment. Without T-cells there was nothing with which to experiment; the virus had not survived. A promising line of research had hit a roadblock.

Meanwhile, on the clinical front the AIDS dilemma took a quantum leap. Clinicians observed that for every patient diagnosed with AIDS, there were 10 times as many who had conditions that seemed to be related. These patients did not fit the strict CDC definition of AIDS, which included only those patients with *Pneumocystis carinii* or

Kaposi's sarcoma who were previously healthy individuals.

These new patients had any of a number of conditions that did not fit that description, but which appeared frequently in high-risk individuals and were accompanied by some degree of damage to the immune system. These included persistent swollen glands, chronic diarrhea, weight loss, night sweats, depression, and loss of hair. Some of these patients would go on to develop AIDS. Others would have chronic conditions similar to those observed in AIDS patients. Few would improve in condition.

It became clear to the epidemiologists at the Centers for Disease Control that AIDS was a more complex disease than had been originally presumed. It was obvious that the definition of AIDS should be expanded to include some of these new patients with AIDS-related conditions. The *Morbidity and Mortality Weekly Report* published the new case definition for AIDS in its August 5, 1983, report.

No longer would a patient have to have Kaposi's sarcoma or *Pneumocystis carinii* to be diagnosed with AIDS. Since the key to the disease seemed to be immune deficiency, the Centers for Disease Control described AIDS as "a reliably diagnosed disease that is at least moderately indicative of an underlying cellular immunodeficiency in a person who has had no known cause of underlying cellular immunodeficiency."[11]

Thus the definition of AIDS was expanded. The key to the diagnosis was immune deficiency. But how to draw the line? What was the key between a diagnosis of the less onerous "AIDS-related conditions" and the more drastic diagnosis of AIDS?

The question persists to this day. In 1983 the definition of AIDS was evolving. Patients with conditions that were related to AIDS but not severe enough to diagnose as AIDS (even under the expanded definition) were referred to by a number of terms. These included "pre-AIDS," "AIDS-related conditions" and "AIDS-related complex." Today this group is lumped together under the term "AIDS-related complex," known as ARC.

The line between AIDS-related complex and AIDS is indistinct. A diagnosis of AIDS in the final analysis relies on the clinical judgment of the individual physician. In general, AIDS-related complex is characterized by non-life-threatening infections, and AIDS is characterized by life-threatening infections. In short, AIDS is a designation of inevitability. This has been reinforced with the frequent use of the modifier "full-blown" as in "full-blown AIDS." This differs from AIDS-related complex (ARC), which indicates that there is a possibility that the patient will survive indefinitely, yet suffer from chronic illness.

One of the conditions diagnosed under the general umbrella of ARC is lymphadenopathy syndrome (LAS), which is characterized by severely swollen glands. The recognition that there was a connection between LAS and AIDS was helpful to the French effort to isolate a new virus and identify it as the probable cause of AIDS.

Dr. Luc Montagnier of the Pasteur Institute was performing a variation of an experiment that had turned out unsuccessfully for Dr. Robert Gallo. Dr. Gallo was attempting to prove that there was a retrovirus present in the T-cells of AIDS patients. So he isolated some T-cells from the blood of patients with AIDS and attempted to culture them for several weeks before checking for the retrovirus. The cells died in the interim.

Dr. Montagnier had been approached with some tissue from a patient with lymphadenopathy syndrome. He isolated T-cells from the lymph node, cultured them in fluid, then checked for the presence of a retrovirus in 22 days, about half the time Dr. Gallo had waited. Significantly, tests confirmed that a retrovirus was present.

Dr. Montagnier's methodological caution did not allow him to presume that he had found the AIDS virus. Other human retroviruses had been identified before and, until he knew differently, Montagnier assumed that one of the previously identified retroviruses was causing the positive outcome. The most common of these was the HTLV-I, the human cancer virus which had been originally identified by Dr. Gallo. Montagnier asked Gallo to send him some chemicals that reacted specifically to HTLV-I.

Dr. Montagnier was pleasantly surprised that the chemicals, which reacted only to HTLV-I, did not react to this retrovirus. He concluded that he had isolated a new human retrovirus. Since it had been cultured from a patient with lymphadenopathy syndrome, the retrovirus was called lymphadenopathy-associated virus, or LAV.

The excitement that this news caused in the scientific community was considerable. Identifying a virus as the cause of AIDS would be a tremendous breakthrough. Unfortunately, the investigation that had held out so much promise quickly faded, as Montagnier was unable to keep the virus alive. It seemed as though this virus, LAV, needed a supply of new T-cells in order to survive.

While Dr. Montagnier and others in France were identifying a retrovirus associated with LAS, Dr. Gallo had also isolated and photographed a new human retrovirus that was associated with AIDS, but he refused to publish his findings. He realized that association between this virus and AIDS did not prove cause and effect. So he set his sights on fulfilling the exacting requirements of Koch's postulate.

Robert Koch was a German bacteriologist who won the Nobel Prize in 1905. He established a set of standards that modern medical investigators continue to use to prove causality. In order to satisfy Koch's postulate, scientists would have to recover the virus from infected individuals, grow it in the laboratory, infect a healthy specimen, cause the syndrome, and ultimately recover the virus from the previously healthy subject.

At this stage the idea of experimentation with live subjects (i.e., an animal model) was not yet possible due to the inability to grow the virus on a large scale in a laboratory setting. Until the virus could be plentifully reproduced, it could not be subjected to the kind of experimentation that would prove that it was the cause of AIDS. Frustrated by this inability, Dr. Gallo took the virus that had been isolated from AIDS patients and put it in the freezer.

The public's widespread sense of urgency was becoming a near sense of emergency. Dry statistical measurements did not capture the human tragedy that was taking place day by day with victims of AIDS. Some truly horrid stories began to filter out of the high-risk communities, most notably urban male homosexuals. There were stories of AIDS victims who had experienced an entire collapse of their social network. People were ruined financially, physically, emotionally, and socially. In some cases AIDS patients were shunned by health care workers, who left food trays at the door of the hospital room. In some cases families shunned the victims of AIDS, leaving them to die alone. Support groups were formed in hard-hit cities. Virginia Apuzzo, of the National Gay Task Force, said, "We've visited the sick and buried the dead, and we did it not just because it had to be done, but also because nobody else would do it." Morticians sometimes refused to embalm the bodies of AIDS patients.

Meanwhile, the French had published in May 1983 photographs of the virus occupying and killing the T-helper cell.[12] It became apparent that Dr. Montagnier and Dr. Gallo had been frustrated scientifically because the AIDS virus killed the T-helper cell. If a cell could be developed in which the AIDS virus could grow, then it could be scientifically manipulated.

In late 1983 Dr. Mkulas Popovic, an associate of Dr. Gallo, solved this dilemma by developing a cell in which the virus could grow. This was done by taking T-cells from the blood of healthy humans and developing mutant strains. One strain proved to be a type in which the virus could grow but the host cell could live.[13]

Medical investigators had a medium in which to grow the virus, and Dr. Gallo's laboratory was then able to quickly develop tests that accurately identified the presence of antibodies specific to the new retrovirus. This was done by applying standardized procedures to the blood of AIDS patients and devising reliable indications of antibodies to this new virus, which they referred to as HTLV-III.

HTLV-III stands for "human T-cell lymphotropic virus, type III." This acronym can be understood by examining its components. "H"—it invades humans. "T"—it attacks the T-cells. "L"—it is lymphotropic, meaning it produces a predictable outcome in invaded cells. "V"—it is a virus. "Type 3"—it is the third human retrovirus discovered (following HTLV-I and HTLV-II).

In January 1984 Dr. Gallo was prepared to test the hypothesis that AIDS was caused by this new human retrovirus, since he now had the ability to grow the virus in quantity and a test to determine the presence of antibodies. He requested coded blood samples from the Centers for Disease Control. The CDC provided samples from AIDS patients, along with samples from "controls"—patients who did not have AIDS—in a "blind code" so Gallo and his associates could not tell which were which. If Dr. Gallo's hypothesis was correct, the AIDS patients' blood would test positively for the presence of antibodies, while the control samples would test negatively.

When the samples were run and the code revealed, Dr. Gallo's hypothesis proved correct. Although this did not completely fulfill the strict requirements of Koch's postulate, which is the scientific formula for proving cause and effect, a landmark breakthrough had occurred. Dr. Gallo submitted these findings to the medical journal *Science* on March 30, 1984. Gallo's reports were accepted for publication on April 19, 1984.

On April 24, 1984, Margaret Heckler, Secretary of Health and Human Services, announced that the probable cause of AIDS had been discovered and a means of mass-producing the suspected causative agent, a new virus, had been developed. The ability to grow virus and test for antibodies soon led to confirmation by French investigators that this new human retrovirus was the cause of AIDS.

The AIDS virus has been called by three names. The Americans refer to it as HTLV-III, as named by Dr. Gallo. The French call it LAV, or lymphadenopathy-associated virus. This is because it was isolated by the French from some tissue of a patient with lymphadenopathy syndrome. In Australia and other parts of the world it has been called ARV, or AIDS-associated retrovirus. For simplicity's sake, we will refer to it as the AIDS virus. (A further explanation of the variants of the AIDS virus will be found on pages 185–186).

Throughout 1984 and early 1985, a number of investigations confirmed the association between the AIDS virus and AIDS. Dr. Gallo had partially fulfilled Koch's postulate by conclusively proving that the AIDS virus could be recovered from AIDS patients and grown in the laboratory. However, to fulfill the exacting requirements of Koch's postulate the virus would have to be "transmitted," i.e., taken from infected individuals, injected into healthy specimens, seen to cause the syndrome, and recovered from previously healthy specimens. Dr. Gallo collaborated with Dr. Harvey Alter, Director of the Blood Bank at the National Institutes of Health (NIH), who had been investigating transfusion-associated AIDS.

Alter took large volumes of cell-free plasma from human AIDS patients and injected it intravenously into chimpanzees. Chimpanzees were used because they had no known natural occurrence of an AIDS-like illness. Over time, many of the recipient chimps developed AIDS virus antibodies, and the virus was recovered from their blood. In some of the infected primates, lymphadenopathy developed and laboratory abnormalities appeared resembling those seen in humans with AIDS.

After Alter's findings were published (indicating "successful" transmission), most investigators were content that Koch's postulate had been satisfied. Ethically, the criteria could never be fulfilled with human subjects, but consensus would uphold the chimpanzee model as an acceptable substitute. An etiologic (causative) relationship had been established between the AIDS virus and the dread disease.

The brilliant investigators who discovered the cause of AIDS are truly heroic individuals. Their imagination, methodology, persistence, and cooperation make the race to discover the cause of AIDS one of the most instructive scientific investigative stories of modern times. But identifying a cause is only an arrival at the starting line of a much longer race—the development of vaccine or treatment for AIDS. Although the killer virus had finally been exposed, science had only identified the opponent, not developed a strategy to defeat it.

By the time the cause of AIDS was announced, in April 1984, more than 5,000 cases had been diagnosed and more than 2,000 people had died. Since that time, an international research effort of almost unparalleled proportions has taken place. In the four-month period between January and April 1985, for example, 582 articles in the scientific literature were published about the AIDS virus. In spite of these intensive efforts, the average life span of an AIDS patient remained the same—18 months following diagnosis.

As of September 1985, more than 13,000 AIDS cases have been diagnosed in this country, with over 6,000 deaths. The pattern continues. AIDS afflicts the young in great numbers and remains incurable. Because of this, AIDS victims suddenly have had a peculiar set of circumstances thrust upon them.

For those in high-risk groups, unrelenting reports of diseased and dying members of their community suggest that nearly everyone is at risk. The fact that any sexual contact in the past few years represents a possible source of infection contributes to a general sense of vulnerability on the part of high-risk group members. For this reason many members of high-risk groups live in a state of fear, watching for the first signs of AIDS or ARC.

The line between AIDS and ARC is indistinct. Because of this, patients who are told they are suffering from ARC have to cope with the stress of uncertainty. There is no way to tell which patients will go on to develop AIDS. ARC patients have no control over their fate. Johnny Greene, a writer with ARC, writes:

> Conceivably, I may avoid a full-blown case, but within the past years I have buried so many friends and acquaintances with AIDS and have been exposed so constantly that I too am one of its victims—emotionally, if not physically. As such I live in an eerie limbo, like a prisoner on death row who keeps getting reprieves. And after a year I have asked the question "Doctor, do I have AIDS?" so often it is now a refrain that sums up my whole life. Each morning I wonder if this is the day purple spots indicating Kaposi's sarcoma will appear on my legs. Frequently I set my alarm clock for odd hours to wake and see if I am sleeping through a deep night sweat. Daily I search my neck and body for swollen lymph glands. I monitor my weight and each ounce I lose throws me into a tailspin, doubling my doubt and uncertainty.*

In addition to growing anxiety about their own condition ARC patients have to consider the fears of loved ones. The fear of contracting the AIDS virus prevents loved ones from giving the kind of full support usually given to the seriously ill. The ARC patient also has to reexamine his or her intimate contacts. Who should be told? What should they be told? In addition to this, ARC patients become protective of their medical condition among coworkers. The job becomes important: financially, because of health insurance coverage, and also because it provides continuity in a world that has been severely disrupted.

ARC patients in some cases fight an imaginary battle of will with the disease, anthropomorphizing it. Johnny Greene writes: "Gradually as I reshape my life because of

* Johnny Greene. A writer fights a faceless enemy and learns to live with fear. *People* Magazine June 17, 1985, p. 49

AIDS, I reach an accommodation, an understanding with my enemy. I flatter myself in thinking I have fought AIDS to a standoff in a yearlong mano-a-mano duel. More important, at times I have forced him to show his hand, and I have forced myself to look, to see exactly what I can expect if he wins."*

ARC patients, at best, live with chronic illness. If their condition worsens and they are diagnosed as having full-blown AIDS, the news is devastating. In other patients with terminal illness, the shock and depression often give way to denial. This is not as accessible a psychological mechanism for AIDS patients. The facts are well known. Nearly half of the people who have been diagnosed with AIDS are dead. This fraction has remained nearly constant since its discovery and shows no sign of abating. The amount of attention the media has given to the deadly nature of the disease makes it difficult for an AIDS patient to find a refuge from this reality.

Patients with AIDS are vulnerable in a number of ways. Due to the results of opportunistic infections they may experience dizziness, fatigue, loss of orientation, and loss of memory. Daily chores become difficult and in some cases impossible. They often require the aid of support groups such as the Gay Men's Health Crisis in New York. Volunteers help with buying food and, eventually, dressing and bathing.

AIDS patients also have to cope with an altered physical appearance. Many experience severe weight loss. There are examples of men six feet tall weighing less than 100 pounds at death. This has often been described as a general "wasting away." Other physical changes are the development of darkened patches of skin and purple or red lesions (in patients with Kaposi's sarcoma). AIDS patients who were previously proud of their physical appearance cannot bear to look in mirrors at themselves. Others use a mirror briefly each day to apply makeup to their lesions.

---

*Greene, p. 49.

Another common experience of AIDS patients is the total collapse of their professional and financial status. AIDS patients often keep the knowledge of their condition from their employers for as long as possible. Sooner or later employers find out. This happens either because they become suspicious and demand to know or, more often, because the patient cannot perform at the job in a consistent manner. Healthy AIDS patients have been fired from their jobs in some cases. Cases such as these are currently being challenged in court. In rare cases employers make an effort to work out some sort of arrangement so that an AIDS patient can stay employed for as long as possible. The disease becomes so debilitating that eventually the AIDS patient no longer can work.

Loss of employment is a severe blow for two reasons. It means that a patient no longer has an income, at a time when financial needs are great. Perhaps more significantly it means loss of health insurance unless the employer takes the most unusual step of continuing to pay for it. AIDS patients must go through the bureaucracy necessary to qualify for many state and federal programs. To do this, they must divest themselves of most of their resources, sometimes necessitating a move out of a comfortable living situation into a small, depressing living space.

In some cases AIDS patients have nowhere to live while they wait to die. In one publicized example in Baltimore, a 32-year-old AIDS patient was rejected by his former lover, his two brothers, and discharged from the hospital. He was taken in by a woman who rejected him after a weekend stay, fearful that her children might become infected. He stayed with another couple for two weeks, and they asked him to leave, having been pressured by threatening phone calls. He was in a commune home as of August 1985, waiting to die. The social worker who was assigned to help him get his Social Security benefits was so afraid of becoming infected she would only talk with him by phone.

AIDS patients have a complex set of needs. Because medical science is at present helpless to save them, a great deal of the support comes in the form of counseling. In areas hard hit by AIDS, well-organized programs of community volunteer support, support groups for patients and their loved ones, and individual counseling try to help affected individuals adjust to the reality of terminal illness.

Terminally ill patients can generally count on their families for unconditional support in coping with their situation, but AIDS patients often have an ambiguous and strained relationship with their families. The family members are hit with the news of a family member's fatal illness and simultaneously fear contracting the disease themselves. Many of the victims of AIDS have been homosexuals with a degree of separation and alienation from their primary families. In one study of gay AIDS patients, 80 % had not told their primary family of their homosexuality. In these cases the siblings and parents have to deal with a topic that has previously been suppressed, at the same time they are anticipating the death of the young family member.

Other AIDS patients have had to confess to drug addiction or promiscuity. There is an inevitable anger on the part of the family members for not having been informed and, presumably, being locked out of a potentially life-saving role. In some families siblings know more than parents and there is focus on suspicion, guilt, and anger instead of compassion for the victim.

Family members of AIDS patients have peculiar stresses as well. They are often reluctant to tell others of the situation because of the prejudice many have towards AIDS patients. Thus they have to cope without the normal support network usually afforded family members of terminally ill patients. Parents whose son or daughter contracts AIDS have to cope with the realization that they will outlive one of their progeny.

As AIDS patients proceed toward the terminal stages of the illness, they often experience hallucinations and prolonged comas. In moments of clarity they have to make estate arrangements and in some cases participate in the planning of their own memorial services. The illness, suffering, and eventual death of an AIDS patient epitomizes the word "tragedy." It is impossible to understand why a young, vital life has been extinguished. To have experienced, even in the most remote fashion, a death by AIDS is to be forever changed.

CHAPTER 6 REFERENCES

1. CDC. Prevention of acquired immune deficiency syndrome (AIDS): Report of inter-agency recommendations, Morbid Mortal Weekly Rep. 32:101, 1983.
2. Downon E, Penalba C, Wolff Metal, AIDS in a Haitian couple living in Paris (letter) Lancet 1:1040, 1983.
3. Harris C, Small C B, Klein R S, et al. Immunodeficiency in female sexual partners of men with the acquired immunodeficiency syndrome. N Engl J Med 308:1181, 1983.
4. Oleske J, Minnefor A, Cooper R, et al. Immune deficiency syndrome in children. JAMA 249:2345, 1983.
5. Rubenstein A, Sicklick M, Gupta A, et al. Acquired immunodeficiency with reversed T4IT8 ratios in infants born to promiscuous and drug-addicted mothers. JAMA 249:2350, 1983.
6. Pape J W, Liautaud B, Thomas F, et al. Characteristics of the acquired immunodeficiency syndrome (AIDS) in Haiti, N Engl J Med 309: 945, 1983.
7. Malebranche R, Arnoux E, Guerin J M, et al. Acquired immunodeficiency syndrome with sever gastrointestinal manifestations in Haiti. Lancet 2:873, 1983.
8. WHO. Summary of meetings on AIDS, Geneva, Switzerland, November 22-25, 1983.
9. Kornfeld H, Van de Stowe R A, Lange M, et al. T-lymphocyte subpopulations in homosexual men. N Engl J Med 307:729, 1982.
10. Gill J C, Menitove J E, Wheeler D, et al. Generalized lymphadenopathy and T-cell abnormalities in hemophilia. A. J Pediatr 103:18, 1983.

11. CDC. Update: Acquired immunodeficiency syndrome (AIDS)–United States. Morbid Mortal Weekly Rep 32:389, 1983.

12. Barre-Sinoussi F, Chermann J C, Rey F, et al. Isolation of a T-lymphotropic retrovirus from a patient at risk for acquired immune deficiency syndrome (AIDS). Science 220:868, 1983.

13. Gallo R C, Shaw G M, Markham P D. Etiology of AIDS. In *AIDS: Etiology, Diagnosis, Treatment and Prevention*. De Vita VT, Hellman S, Rosenberg S A (eds). J. B. Lippincott Company, New York, p. 31-54, 1985.

7

Millions May Die

The investigative work of Drs. Gallo, Montagnier, Rosenbaum, and others provided medical science with a true starting point for in-depth study of AIDS virus infection. As the outbreak of AIDS took place in 1982 and 1983, clinicians noticed that a number of patients were appearing with various evidences of immune suppression not always severe enough to diagnose as AIDS. With the development of a blood test, the definite link between "AIDS-related conditions" (finally standardized in 1984 as AIDS-related complex) and AIDS could be made.

The International Conference on AIDS, held in Atlanta in April 1985, gave the world's top AIDS investigators an opportunity to exchange information. By this time AIDS had been observed in all six major continents. Consensus had formed on a number of issues. First, AIDS and ARC patients have been infected with the same agent—the AIDS virus. Second, a large number of symptomless individuals have also been infected with the virus. Third, most individuals remain symptomless for at least a year following infection. Fourth, a large number (perhaps more than half) will develop no signs of AIDS or ARC for at least five years following infection. Fifth, the AIDS virus can be transmitted heterosexually as well as through homosexual contact and sharing of infected blood.

What happens to people infected with the AIDS virus? This is best addressed in two parts. First is a description of the two generally recognized states other than full-blown AIDS resulting from infection: *symptomless carrier* and *AIDS-related complex*. Following this is a projection of what the chances are of being in one state as opposed to another during the first five years of infection.

Symptomless Carriers

Dr. James Curran has conclusively shown that AIDS virus infection is persistent and may be totally symptomless.[1,2] Curran and CDC coworkers traced cases of transfusion-associated full-blown AIDS to infected donors who were free of overt manifestations when they gave the deadly blood. Follow-up investigations revealed over 90% had live AIDS virus circulating in their bloodstreams.

Other studies have recovered infectious AIDS virus from the tears, saliva, semen, and urine of symptomless individuals.[3-6] AIDS virus infiltrates the eyes, brain, lungs, liver, spleen, kidneys, and other organs of infected persons, including those who remain symptomless.

Nearly all infected individuals will remain symptomless for the first year following infection. Unfortunately, less than 1% of the symptomless carriers will be identified by blood testing this year in America. Symptomless carriers who are unaware of their infection (and they number more than 1 million) are putting every sexual contact at risk. Symptomless individuals can transmit AIDS contagion for at least five years and probably much longer. This is why the AIDS virus spreads so rapidly.

The virus can be transmitted from symptomless mother

to infant.[7] It is possible for a husband to unknowingly infect his wife, who can then transmit the infection to their infant. A tragic illustration of this is the case of the Burk family of Cresson, Pennsylvania. Patrick Burk is a hemophiliac and received the AIDS virus from some blood concentrate that was used to treat him. He passed the virus on to his wife, Lauren, and from her it infected their son, Dwight. Today, all three are suffering from AIDS or ARC.

In addition to the possibility of infecting their sexual partners, symptomless carriers may have their lives complicated in other ways. The AIDS virus blood test is being considered as a marital screen and as a prerequisite for insurance (see Chapter 9). The military plans to use the AIDS virus blood test as a screen, and the health care and other professions may restrict infected individuals as well.

A symptomless carrier is a person whose medical condition is under a constant threat. Otherwise healthy AIDS-virus-positive individuals may at any time suffer a replicative attack and suffer immune system damage. The fact that the virus may be triggered by such events as surgery, pregnancy, or serious illness means that symptomless carriers of the AIDS virus live in a permanently precarious medical state. Although it appears that more than half of the individuals infected with the AIDS virus will remain symptomless for the first five years, their long-range prognosis is unknown. There are indications that future complications of AIDS virus infection may include a variety of cancers (primarily blood malignancies) and neurological disorders. Because of their potential infectivity to others and their cloudy personal medical outlook, even those fortunate individuals who remain symptomless for five years can be included among the victims of the deadly AIDS virus.

AIDS-Related Complex

AIDS-related complex (ARC) is, in a sense, a lesser form of AIDS. In addition to being infectious, ARC patients show signs of an immune system that has been attacked and damaged but not incapacitated.

Individuals are generally diagnosed as having ARC if they test positively on the AIDS virus blood test and show two or more of the following manifestations: persistent fever (100° for three months or more), persistent swollen glands, weight loss of more than 10% or 15 pounds, diarrhea, fatigue, or night sweats. The AIDS virus has demonstrated the ability to invade the brain and central nervous system.[8,9] This can cause loss of memory, tremors, seizures and speech impairment in people with ARC.

There are actually more than 50 clinical manifestations of ARC. People who suffer from ARC live with chronic, recurring illness. Further, they evidence many of the psychological stresses and social consequences of AIDS patients. Some of the people with ARC will eventually develop full-blown AIDS and die.[10,11] *Pneumocystis carinii* or Kaposi's sarcoma in an ARC patient establishes the diagnosis of full-blown AIDS. ARC sufferers are vigilant for the telltale purple or reddish spots indicating Kaposi's sarcoma or the suffocating dry cough signifying *Pneumocystis* pneumonia. ARC patients who live on a regular basis with irrefutable evidence of AIDS virus infection and attack often fall prey to the anxiety and depression well described previously by Johnny Greene. Because the CDC does not require health care professionals to report ARC, the number of ARC sufferers will continue to be inexact, with current estimates ranging from 50,000 to 200,000. Best available information indicates that 25% of an infected group will develop ARC (without developing AIDS) within five years of infection.[12] However, the likely conversion percentage for years six and beyond will not be accurately known for quite some time.

Five-Year Projection

One of the most important questions relating to AIDS virus infection is, "What percent of an infected population will eventually develop full-blown AIDS?" This has been described by Dr. Michael Lange of St. Luke's Hospital in New York as "the million-dollar question."

Unfortunately, there is little data currently available on this important subject. This is because in order to make a calculation it is necessary to study a group of infected individuals over a period of several years. Because the blood test for the AIDS virus was only developed in 1984, "longitudinal studies" (with a group over time) could only be performed by analyzing blood samples that were stored from other investigations.

The most frequently cited figure estimating the conversion from AIDS virus infection to full-blown AIDS was included in the March 1985 Food and Drug Administration bulletin on AIDS: "5 to 19 percent of (infected) homosexual men developed AIDS within 2-5 years (of infection)."[11] The data on which these figures are based come from the following studies.

Goedert and coworkers[13,14] followed 48 infected homosexual male residents of New York City and Washington, D.C., for more than two years and found that 9 (19%) developed full-blown AIDS. Melbye and associates[15] found that of 22 infected volunteers from a gay organization in Denmark, 2 (9%) developed the full-blown syndrome over a 14-month observation period. Since all these men were infected when the study began, the average time lag between infection and the development of AIDS cannot be established from these data. Jaffee and others[12] found 31 homosexual men seen in a San Francisco City clinic who were infected with the AIDS virus between 1978 and 1980. From this group of 31, 2 (6%) developed full-blown AIDS and 8 (25%) developed ARC over an average follow-up period of 61 months.

Mathur-Wagh and coinvestigators[10,16] reported on a group of 42 homosexual men from New York City with swollen glands. Ten (24%) met the CDC surveillance criteria for full-blown AIDS within a 40-month follow-up period. The average time between the onset of enlarged glands and the diagnosis of full-blown AIDS was 24 months. CDC investigator Fishbein[11] reported 5 (6%) of 78 homosexual or bisexual men followed for generalized gland swelling developed AIDS 5 to 25 months after the change in gland size. Groopman and associates[17] studied homosexual men in Boston and found that 6 (8%) of 78 with swollen glands developed full-blown AIDS. One must be aware of the limitations of these studies. All of them involved men who already had manifestations of ARC. Thus they yield an unrepresentative view of the consequences of AIDS virus infection in a population over time.

Insight into the question of the conversion time between infection and the development of full-blown AIDS (also referred to as the "incubation period") comes from a study of hemophiliacs by Eyster and collaborators.[18] Stored blood samples were retrieved and analyzed for AIDS virus antibodies. Among 30 hemophiliacs that were positive, 10 (33%) were infected during 1979–1981, 12 (40%) during 1982, and 10 (33%) during 1983–1984. Seven of 10 who were infected for more than three years had developed generalized swollen glands. In contrast, only 1 of the 9 patients who were infected for less than two years had enlarged glands. Among the 11 patients who were infected for two to three years, 1 had abnormal glands. Two (10%) of the 21 patients infected for more than two years had died of full-blown AIDS. These findings suggest the first manifestations of disease appear two years after infection, and by three to five years many of those infected will develop AIDS or ARC.

Additional insight into the question of conversion time between infection and the development of manifestations of AIDS or ARC has been provided by Dr. Anthony Fauci,[19] a director of the National Institute of Allergy and Infectious Diseases. Dr. Fauci is heading much of the NIH clinical research on possible treatments for AIDS. His work indicates that the average incubation time varies according to the type of transmission. Dr. Fauci has estimated the average time lag between infection and the *first recognizable signs or symptoms of AIDS or ARC.* (N.B. The average time for the development of full-blown AIDS will obviously be longer.) People who are infected sexually begin to develop clinical manifestations in 12 to 14 months, intravenous drug users in two years, transfusion recipients and hemophiliacs in two to five years, and infants in a matter of months.

Drs. Goedert and Blattner of the National Cancer Institute recently interpreted the available data and described the annual "attack rate" of full-blown AIDS in infected individuals as dynamic, increasing from virtually zero in the first year to 7% annually during the third and fourth years of infection. Recent data suggest sometime after the fourth or fifth year following infection the annual AIDS incidence rate will decline. Should this prove correct, it is possible that less than 1% will convert at the end of year one, 5% at the end of year two, 10% after year three, and 20% by the end of year five.

The AIDS virus began infecting Americans in great numbers starting in early 1980. Thus the data we are currently collecting are only indicative of how the virus acts in a population over this rather short time frame. The prognosis for AIDS-virus-positive people is currently under study; the Department of Health and Human Services included $1 million in its 1986 budget proposal to investigate this question. All individuals infected with the AIDS virus have legitimate concern about their medical future.

How Many Americans Are Infected?

Although only a percentage of a population infected with the AIDS virus will develop AIDS or ARC within five years of infection, every person infected has an ambiguous medical outlook, both short and long range. It is only natural to wonder, "How many Americans are infected with the AIDS virus?"

As of the middle of 1985, most knowledgeable scientists were estimating 1 million or more. Dr. James Mason,

Acting Assistant Secretary for Health of the Department of Health and Human Services, said in late July that it was likely 1 million Americans had been infected.[20] Dr. Michael Gottlieb of the UCLA School of Medicine put the number between 500,000 and 1 million.[20] Dr. Dani Bolognesi, of the Duke University Medical Center put the figure at 2 million.[20]

These figures are all educated estimates. No definitive number will be known unless mandatory blood screening of the adult population is implemented. Since federal efforts in this country will identify less than 1% of the symptomless carriers of the AIDS virus this year, all American data will involve a degree of unreliability. However, there are some counting methods by which we can infer the probable extent of infection.

Studies of sexually active urban homosexual men indicate a tremendous increase of infection over the last several years. San Francisco blood samples from men attending a clinic for sexually transmitted diseases showed 1% infection in 1978, 25% in 1980, and 65% in 1984.[21] Current estimates indicate infection in sexually active homosexual men in San Francisco and New York to be 70–90 percent. Other cities have shown an explosive growth rate of infection, Denver rising from 10% in 1978 to 49% in 1984 and Pittsburgh growing from 10% in 1983 to 28% in 1984.[22]

How many homosexual men nationwide are currently infected with the AIDS virus? Drs. Fischinger and Bolognesi suggest that 55% of American homosexual men are infected in areas where AIDS is epidemic.[23] Since much of the data used in this survey was collected in urban areas, the actual percentage is likely to be lower. It is reasonable to postulate national infection in the middle of 1985 to be in the 10–15% range. According to Kinsey's historical estimate that 10% of adult males are homosexual, this would calculate (with 160 million American adults) to 800,000 to 1.2 million in this group alone.

Intravenous drug users are also infected in great numbers. AIDS virus infection rose from 29% among intravenous drug users attending a clinic in Queens, New York, in 1981–82 to 87% in a similar clinic sampled in Manhattan in 1984.[11-22,24] Fischinger and Bolognesi[23] estimated infection among drug users nationwide to be as high as 87%. It is estimated that there are 400,000 regular users of intravenous drugs and an additional half million intermittent users. If even 25% of the regular users and an additional 10% of the intermittent users are infected, there would be 150,000 infected intravenous drug users at present.

It is worth noting that 20% of intravenous drug users are female and one-third of those surveyed admit to prostitution as a means of supporting their drug habit.[25] This means that there may be 9,000 or more infected prostitutes from this group.

Hemophiliacs have also been infected with the AIDS virus. Infection among hemophiliacs and transfusion recipients (prior to April 1985) was also significant. Fischinger and Bolognesi suggest infection among hemophiliacs to be at least 72% nationally.[23] However, it is safer to project that half of the 15,000 hemophiliacs nationwide are infected. New infection among transfusion recipients and hemophiliacs has been nearly eliminated due to federal action beginning in April, 1985, to screen all blood donated. The number of transfusion recipients infected by blood donated before March 1985 is difficult to estimate.

Infection among recent (post-1978) immigrants from Haiti and central Africa is significant as well. A 1985 report estimated that 40% of the roughly 100,000 who immigrated from Haiti since 1978 were infected with the AIDS virus.[23] There is no data available on central African immigrants. However, since AIDS virus infection is more prevalent in central Africa than Haiti, it would not be surprising to find a comparable or higher percentage infected from this group. It is reasonable to speculate that there are at least 40,000 recent immigrants from these areas infected with the AIDS virus.

Based on these calculations, it appears that there are between 1 and 1.5 million people from these high-risk groups infected with the AIDS virus. With even a conservative estimate of the extent of infection beyond these groups, it is clear that AIDS virus infection represents a national public health problem of staggering proportions.

Do American Heterosexuals Have Anything To Fear?

How Many Are Already Infected?

The story of the heterosexual spread of AIDS and the AIDS virus in America has been one of the most "underreported" aspects of the epidemic to date. This is due in some degree to a semantic manipulation on the part of the Centers for Disease Control, which reports the number of AIDS cases in various categories.

See the table below:

AIDS Cases as of September 23, 1985

	Men	Women
Homosexual or Bisexual	9,711	0
Intravenous Drug Users	1,790	459
Transfusion Recipients	121	87
Hemophiliacs	89	4
Heterosexuals	15	118
Others	627	195
	12,353	863

Of the 13,216 adult AIDS cases reported through Sept. 1985, 9,711 (73.5%) occurred in male homosexuals or bisexuals. The other cases (more than 26.5%) occurred in heterosexuals. The fact that many of these heterosexuals are intravenous drug users should not disguise the fact that more than one-quarter of AIDS cases to date have taken place in heterosexual men and women. A cursory glance at the table would cause the careless reader to interpret heterosexual AIDS as comprising 133 (less than 1%) of the cases.

What does this mean about the likely extent of AIDS

virus infection among American heterosexuals? If the ratio observed in these cases holds true for the current pattern of infected Americans, then there are at least 250,000 infected American heterosexuals in the high-risk groups alone. Since the AIDS virus has been transmitted through heterosexual contact, the spread of infection to other heterosexuals beyond these groups is a foregone conclusion.

African AIDS—A Model of Heterosexual Spread

Information about the spread of AIDS in Africa has some disturbing implications for American heterosexuals. African AIDS began appearing at about the same time as American AIDS. There are some crucial differences between the emerging patterns in the two areas. Between May 1979 and April 1983, 18 previously healthy African patients were hospitalized for full-blown AIDS. Their illnesses were characterized by either opportunistic infection, Kaposi's sarcoma, or both. Ten of them died by the end of 1983. The study, reported initially in the *New England Journal of Medicine,*[26] underscores the significance of their lack of high-risk factors (as observed in American AIDS patients). None had any history of intravenous drug use, homosexuality, or blood transfusion. This was one of the first suggestions that an outbreak of AIDS was taking place in Africa. It also, of course, suggests that the AIDS virus can be spread in populations other than those in American high-risk categories.

A few months later there was another group of African AIDS patients studied,[27] this time from the central African country of Rwanda. A questionnaire circulated among health care professionals turned up a group of 17 males and 9 females with AIDS. Once again, previously noted American high-risk characteristics did not hold. The three factors that did correlate were *upper-middle-class status, urban residence, and heterosexual promiscuity.*

Further investigation shows an explosion of AIDS virus infection and an unfolding epidemic of AIDS cases in central Africa, closely linked to heterosexual promiscuity. In a study of prostitutes from Rwanda in 1984, 88% were found to be infected with the AIDS virus. A study of men who frequently are customers of prostitutes showed that 28% were infected.[28] Studies of the adult populations in general show that 8% or more of Zaire adults are infected,[29] 21% in Kenya,[29] 10% in Rwanda, and 23% in Zambia. The disease has appeared in a total of 20 African countries including Burundi, Tanzania, and Angola. The AIDS virus has obviously spread rapidly in central Africa in the past few years. (See Figure 7–1.) Further, heterosexual contact appears to be the most prevalent form of transmission, with prostitute contact facilitating the spread.

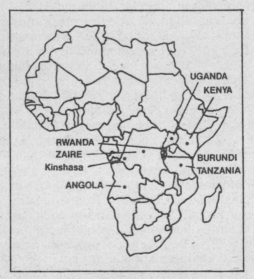

Figure 7-1. African spread.

Is the information in Africa applicable to America? It is plausible to suggest that the main difference between the patterns of African and American AIDS is due to a different starting point. It is clear that urban male homosexuals were the first group infected in significant numbers in the American pattern of spread. Urban gay male communities in the late 1970s and early 1980s were characterized by promiscuity and a relatively "closed" nature (a high proportion of homosexuals to bisexuals). By homosexuals keeping mostly to themselves, AIDS virus infection was contained in the gay population.

Would the American pattern of spread more closely mimic the African pattern if the original portal of entry of the AIDS virus in America was in a promiscuous heterosexual community? Undoubtedly, the signs of such a spread are currently visible in our society.

AIDS as a Sexually Transmitted Disease

The explosive growth of AIDS virus infection in America, Africa, and Haiti strongly resembles the pattern seen in other sexually transmitted diseases. Often referred to as "venereal disease (VD)," sexually transmitted diseases include genital herpes, syphilis, gonorrhea, nonspecific urethritis, genital warts, and hepatitis B. Contagion can be passed by oral-oral, oral-genital, genital-genital, genital-rectal and oral-rectal contact. Figures 7-2, 7-3, and 7-4 suggest the attack rates of several common sexually transmitted diseases.

Figure 7-2 depicts the annual number of cases of gonorrhea and nonspecific urethritis in men reported from clinics in England and Wales. Between 1968-1974 the infection rate of gonorrhea remained relatively stable while the nonspecific urethritis cases doubled. Both gonorrhea and nonspecific urethritis are easily treated with oral antibiotics. Some individuals are successfully treated but are subsequently reinfected.

Figure 7-3 shows an estimated rate of patient consultation

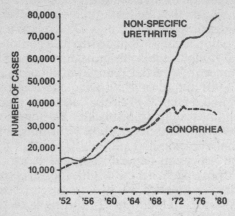

Figure 7-2. Annual number of cases of gonorrhea and non-specific urethritis in men reported from clinics in England and Wales, 1951–1980.

for genital warts seen by physicians in private practice in the United States. The office visits increased over 400% between 1966 and 1982, indicating substantial growth in prevalence. Genital warts are caused by the papilloma virus, which is treatable but difficult to completely eradicate. Successful therapy requires multiple patient consultations.

Figure 7–4 illustrates dramatic growth in patient consultations for genital herpes in the United States. Individuals typically seek medical help for herpes due to genital pain. Between 1966 and 1981 patient visits for genital herpes increased more than 1,000%. The genital herpes virus replicates periodically, producing sores. Genital herpes sufferers are actively shedding infectious virus during periods of viral replication and blister formation. Theoretically, if those infected by genital herpes would abstain during times of viral activity, the attack rate on new individuals would drop precipitously. A recently developed vaccine and the relatively new antiviral agent acyclovir promise to alter the future of genital herpes virus. Unfortunately,

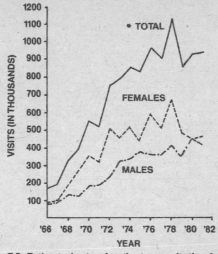

Figure 7-3. Estimated rate of patient consultation for genital warts seen by physicians in private practice, United States, 1966–1982. *Includes visits by patients with gender not stated. (From the National Diseases and Therapeutic Index.)

these medical breakthroughs occurred after 20 million Americans were infected.

If a 1,000% increase in genital herpes over 15 years seems scary, look at Figure 7–5, which charts the number of new AIDS cases among homosexual men diagnosed in each quarter year in America from July 1978 through October 1984. Because of the astronomical increase in reported cases of AIDS between 1982–1984, the top third of the area represents roughly three-fourths of the numbers. Over the 4 years from 1980 to 1984 the number of new cases of full-blown AIDS among homosexual men increased over 10,000%. The AIDS virus has awesome power to replicate and attack within a sexually active community.

One reason for the dramatic increase of AIDS is the absence of curative treatment to reduce the spread of new infection. One way of visualizing this is to contrast it with a curable disease, such as syphilis. Syphilis can be treated in

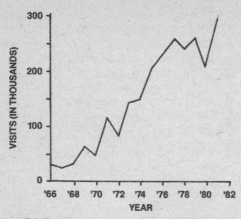

Figure 7-4. Estimated rate of patient consultations for genital herpes seen by physicians in private practice, United States, 1966–1981. (From the National Diseases and Therapeutic Index.)

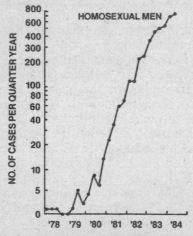

Figure 7-5. Semilogarithmic graph of the number of new U.S. AIDS cases among homosexual men diagnosed in each quarter-year, 1978 to July 1, 1984 (reported as of October 29, 1984).

such a way that the infected individual is no longer contagious. So, for example, if 100 prostitutes in a given city contracted syphilis in a certain month and 80 of them were treated, there would be only 20 who remained infectious. If 100 prostitutes, on the other hand, were infected with the AIDS virus in a given month, all 100 would indefinitely remain infectious.

Prostitutes, both male and female, have long been associated with the rapid spread of sexually transmitted disease. A study of female street prostitutes was done in Colorado Springs[30] which showed that 63% were infected with gonorrhea in a 14-month period. Had they been infected with the AIDS virus they would be forever infectious. In addition to being highly susceptible to sexually transmitted disease, prostitutes have also shown the ability to infect others in great numbers. One study traced nearly one-fourth of all 1976 cases of gonorrhea in Colorado Springs (a city of 200,000) to just 56 prostitutes.[30]

What role do prostitutes play in spreading AIDS virus infection in America? There may be as many as 9,000 infected female prostitutes nationwide who are intravenous drug users and thousands more who do not use intravenous drugs. Male prostitutes are believed to have been instrumental in the Haitian and African spread of the AIDS virus, and may have accelerated the process of American infection by contact with vacationing gay men. American male prostitutes have likely facilitated the spread of AIDS virus infection.

Particularly troubling is the fact that the four cities which have the largest number of AIDS cases—New York, San Francisco, Los Angeles, and Miami—have a tremendous number of out-of-town visitors. Traveling business and professional people who become infected with the AIDS virus by contact with a prostitute can then return to their home area and initiate a chain reaction of AIDS virus infection by unwittingly introducing the AIDS virus into a sexually active subpopulation[25]

In the 1950s a movie was made to try and explain in

simple terms how a nuclear fission reaction develops. A room was filled with a set of mousetraps and Ping Pong balls were placed on each trap. One ball was dropped into the middle of the room, initiating a chain reaction of traps being sprung and balls being set in motion. In a short period of time, nearly all of the traps had been sprung. Once the first ball was dropped, it irrevocably set into motion the process by which the rest would be sprung. Once the process began, there was no turning back. It is logical to wonder in which communities the AIDS virus currently is being similarly spread.

Once the AIDS virus has achieved a portal of entry into a sexually active community, it has shown remarkable ability to infect large percentages of the community. Whatever the exact requirements that are necessary for transmission to take place (explored in greater detail in the next chapter) any virus that can infect three-quarters or more of the sexually active gay populations of New York and San Francisco in less than a decade is infectious indeed.

The "Attack Rate" of the AIDS Virus

One can estimate the attack rate of the AIDS virus in America by utilizing data available on the increase in the number of AIDS cases. It has already been suggested that there is nearly a three-year average time lag between infection and the development of sexually transmitted AIDS. Since roughly three-quarters of the American AIDS cases to date have been due to sexual transmission, one can infer that the pattern of today's AIDS cases is related to the pattern of sexual transmission of three years ago.

Using the assumption of 10% of an infected population developing AIDS at three years following infection, one can infer the following: the 2,200 American AIDS cases reported in homosexual or bisexual men in the year June 1983–May 1984 imply 22,000 infections in the period three years previous (June 1980–May 1981). This kind of mathematical manipulation provides useful insight into the pat-

tern of American spread of AIDS virus infection from
1979–1982:

	Reported Number of AIDS Cases				Estimated Number People Infected	
	Calendar	Cumulative			Calendar	Cumulative
1981	239*	296*		1978	2,500*	3,000*
1982	665	961		1979	7,000	10,000
1983	1,540	2,501		1980	15,000	25,000
1984	4,499	7,100		1981	45,000	70,000

*Although AIDS was officially defined in 1981, reexamina-
tion of medical records caused 4 cases from 1978, 9 from
1979, and 44 from 1980 to be subsequently reclassified as
AIDS. These were added to the 1981 total of 239 to arrive
at the cumulative figure of 296.

This analysis only yields the pattern of infection through
1982. Insights into the infection in 1983 and beyond can be
arrived at inferentially. Dr. Ann Hardy of the Centers for
Disease Control has predicted that there will be 8,500 new
AIDS cases in 1985, an additional 15,000 in 1986, and
27,000 more in 1987. Data through early August supports
the prediction of 8,500 for 1985. There have been over 5,500
new AIDS cases reported in 1985 through September 21,
and the rate of increase above 1984 is rising. There may well
be more than 9,000 by the end of the year.

Dr. Hardy's estimate may prove to be too conservative.
Dr. Thomas Quinn of the National Institutes of Health
predicted in January 1985 that there would be 40,000 AIDS
cases reported in 1985 and 1986.[31] The actual number will
probably be higher than Hardy's estimate of 24,000 and
Quinn's estimate of 40,000. Using the lower figures, our
chart can be extended.

	Number of AIDS Cases			Number of People Infected (estimated)	
	Calendar	Cumulative		Calendar	Cumulative
1981	239	296	1978	2,500	3,000
1982	665	961	1979	7,000	10,000
1983	1,540	2,501	1980	15,000	25,000
1984	4,499	7,100	1981	45,000	70,000
1985 (est.)	8,500	15,600	1982	85,000	155,000
1986 (est.)	15,000	30,600	1983	150,000	305,000
1987 (est.)	27,000	57,000	1984	270,000	575,000

It is worth noting that the estimate of more than 500,000 infected people by the end of 1984 fits well with the comments of epidemiologists who are close to the problem. In June 1985 Dr. James Curran estimated the number of infected Americans to be between 500,000 and 1 million. Others place the numbers higher. The authors believe that by the end of 1985 1.5 million Americans will be infected.

Another useful insight is gained by dividing the number of people estimated to have been infected each year by 12 to see the average per month. This yields:

Estimated Number of People Infected Per Month

Year	Number
1978	200
1979	600
1980	1,250
1981	3,600
1982	7,100
1983	12,500
1984	22,500

An even more detailed analysis can be done utilizing available data on reported and projected AIDS cases broken down semiannually.

1978	Jan.–June	150 per month
1978	Jul.–Dec.	250 per month
1979	Jan.–June	300 per month
1979	Jul.–Dec.	800 per month
1980	Jan.–June	1,700 per month
1980	Jul.–Dec.	2,200 per month
1981	Jan.–June	3,400 per month
1981	Jul.–Dec.	4,000 per month
1982	Jan.–June	5,800 per month
1982	Jul.–Dec.	8,300 per month
1983	Jan.–June	11,100 per month
1983	Jul.–Dec.	14,200 per month
1984	Jan.–June	18,200 per month
1984	Jul.–Dec.	26,700 per month

As 1985 draws to a close, how many people are being infected each day? It is plausible to suggest that the rate of the second half of 1984 has increased by 80%, since this increase appears to hold from one year to the next. This would yield an attack rate of 48,000 per month. This equals 1,600 per day, or nearly one every 60 seconds. We will scale that back due to the hopeful interpretation of data suggesting changing sexual habits in high-risk communities to a conservative estimate of 30,000 per month. This translates into 1,000 every day, or one new infection every 90 seconds.

Should heterosexuals in America be personally concerned about the spread of the AIDS virus? The answer is an emphatic YES. There are already 250,000 infected heterosexuals, and there may be twice or even three times that number. African AIDS presents a compelling model which demonstrates that heterosexual promiscuity can be facilitative for the spread of the AIDS virus. The AIDS virus has a pattern of infection similar to other sexually transmitted diseases. It has demonstrated an attack rate that is increasing exponentially.

What does all of this mean? What is actually happening right now as you read this? Is it possible that one person every minute and a half is being infected with the deadly AIDS virus? Is it possible that every tenth infected person will develop AIDS in three years? Dr. Dani Bolognesi of the Duke University Medical Center said in Congressional testimony of July 22, 1985, "Current estimates indicate that as many as 2 million people in the United States alone have already been infected ... and are therefore at risk for developing the disease. Until preventive measures, such as vaccines, are available, *this number is expected to double each year.*" (Emphasis ours.)

If Dr. Bolognesi's numbers are correct, our calculations are far too conservative. To jump from 2 million infections in July 1985 to 4 million in July 1986 would mean more than 150,000 new individuals would become infected each month. This breaks down to 5,000 per day, or one every 18 seconds. Further, this would mean more than 30 million infected Americans by the end of this decade.

Is this possible? Could AIDS cases double each year until a vaccine is developed (unlikely until 1990 or later)? The growth record of genital herpes infections provides a hint. Genital herpes was almost unheard of in medical journals 30 years ago. The great herpes scare started in the late 1970s. It is estimated in 1985 that 20 million Americans are infected. CDC officials estimate that there are at least 500,000 new cases per year. This phenomenal growth occurred despite the fact that genital herpes creates visible signs of infection within seven days and is much easier to control through voluntary sexual restraint than AIDS virus infection.

It is the time to be truthful about the threat. Twenty million infected Americans would mean 1 million, perhaps 2 million AIDS cases would develop, many of them in young people. Over 90% of the first 4,000 AIDS cases were from 20–49 years old, a pattern that has since continued. As you read this, the AIDS virus is currently infecting 1,000 or more new victims a day. It has gained entrance to various subsets of the heterosexual world, singles bars, nightclubs, college campuses, heterosexual "singles groups," upper-class vacation spots, high-class, expensive "out-call" prostitutes and their customers.

If the AIDS virus is allowed to continue, the day hundreds of thousands or millions of Americans are dying of AIDS may be sooner than most of us could imagine. How can the AIDS threat be stopped? Few people would currently support involuntary measures sponsored by government actions. One academic expert has described a possible approach to the control of sexually transmitted disease, involving mandatory large-scale blood screening followed by the issuance of health identity cards.[32]

A second and more preferable way to slow the growth of infection is through education and a voluntary change in behavior. Only a massive well-organized, powerful, and persuasive education in risk reduction can alter what now appears may be the inevitable infection of millions of Americans during the next few years.

Statistics show that the urban homosexual communities have responded to the AIDS threat by substantially reducing the amount of casual, anonymous sex. One of the best indices of promiscuity is the reported cases of gonorrhea. Gonorrhea is often cited as indicative of trends in sexual activity. In New York City there was a 59% drop in reported cases of gonorrhea between 1980 and 1983.[33] A report at the International Conference on AIDS in Atlanta in April 1985 showed a 70% drop in rectal gonorrhea in San Francisco over the same period of time.[34] Reports from other cities also indicate a tremendous decline in sexually transmitted disease among homosexual men. There has been a 16% drop nationally in reported syphilis cases among men from 1982 to 1984.

Unfortunately, this response was too late to save hundreds of thousands of gay men from being infected with the AIDS virus. It is also unfortunate that while much of the gay community has responded affirmatively, a portion has apparently either rejected or ignored the severity of the threat. Johnny Greene, who is fighting AIDS-related complex, writes in *People* magazine,

> The fear of the virus radically alters my life, and I watch it transform the lives of my friends. Men who once hit the sidewalks and bars nightly retreat into bunkers, suspicious, hostile, and hurt. The bar-scene way of life, with its around-the-clock offer of sexual adventure and escape from reality, has been cut off by AIDS, and gays have yet to find positive alternatives. Other friends carry on with mindless fatalism, hitting the streets at midnight, packing into crowded discos and bars, head banging until dawn on the very lid of death.

A sizable part of the urban gay community has "sobered up." Lifestyles have been drastically altered. "Promiscuity is dead," says Charles Ortleb, publisher of the *New York Native*, the city's leading gay newspaper. But there remains a core of people who are apparently willing to "roll the dice." The AIDS virus is now so prevalent in certain areas that one casual sexual encounter with an anonymous partner today is 100 times more likely to produce infection than the same encounter a few short years ago.

The AIDS virus has already entered a number of heterosexual circles. Will heterosexuals in America also take heed? There is no longer the luxury of time. Will promiscuous heterosexuals have their blood tested voluntarily? Unless this killer is recognized in our midsts, this national state of emergency will become a catastrophe of unimaginable proportions. Will heterosexuals learn from the tragedy that has already occurred? Will they reduce risky sexual behavior, or fatalistically "dance until dawn"?

The party is over. We must snap out of our dream world and face this unpleasant truth. If we do not, it almost surely can destroy us. It is time to "turn out the lights" on a lifestyle of promiscuity—of casual, anonymous sex.

The AIDS virus shows every sign of being just as deadly as the plague during the Middle Ages. We are on a crash course with reality. This is not a practice run. There is no second chance. AIDS may be to the twentieth century what the Black Plague was to the fourteenth century.

The alarm must be sounded, loudly and persuasively. If it is not, the conclusion is inescapable: millions may die.

CHAPTER 7 REFERENCES

1. Feorino PM, Jaffee HW, Palmer E, et al. Transfusion-associated acquired immune deficiency syndrome: Evidence for persistent infection in blood donors, N Engl J Med 312:1293, 1985.
2. Jaffee HW, Feorino PM, Darrow WW, et al. Persistent infection with human T-lymphotropic virus type III/Lymphadenopathy-associated virus in apparently healthy homosexual men. Ann Intern Med 102:627, 1985.
3. Groopman JE, Salahuddin SZ, Sarngadharan MG, et al. HTLV- III in saliva of people with AIDS-related complex and healthy homosexual men at risk for AIDS, Science 226:447, 1984.
4. Ho DD, Schooley RT, Rota TR, et al. HTLV-III in the semen and blood of a healthy homosexual man. Science 226:451, 1984.
5. Salahuddin SZ, Markham PD, Popovic M, et al. Isolation of infectious human T-cell leukemia/lymphotropic virus type III (HTLV-III) from patients with acquired immunodeficiency syndrome (AIDS) or AIDS-related complex (ARC) and from healthy carriers: A study of risk groups and tissue sources. Proc Natl Acad Sci USA 82:5530, 1985.
6. Fujikawa LS, Palestine AY, Nussenblatt RB, et al. Isolation of human T-lymphotropic virus type III from tears of a patient with the acquired immunodeficiency syndrome. Lancet 2:529, 1985.
7. Laurence J, Brun-Vezinet F, Schutzer SF, et al. Lymphadenopathy-associated viral antibodies in AIDS: Immune correlations and definition of a carrier state. N Engl J Med 311:1269, 1984.

8. Gonda MA, Wong-Staal F, Gallo RC. Sequence homology and morphologic similarity of HTLV-III and visnavirus, a pathogenic lentivirus. Science 227:173, 1985.

9. Shaw GM, Harper ME, Hahn BH, et al. HTLV-III infection in brains of children and adults with AIDS encephalopathy. Science 227:177, 1985.

10. Mathur-Wagh U, Spigland I, Sacks HS, et al. Longitudinal study of persistent generalized lympahdenopathy in homosexual men: Relation to acquired immunodeficiency syndrome. Lancet 1:1033, 1984.

11. Fishbein DB, Kaplan JE, Spira TJ, et al. Unexplained lymphadenopathy in homosexual men: A longitudinal study. JAMA 254:930, 1985.

12. Jaffe HW, Darrow WW, Echenberg DF, et al. The acquired immunodeficiency syndrome in a cohort of homosexual men: A six-year follow-up study. Ann Intern Med 103:210, 1985.

13. Goedert JJ, Sarngadharan MG, Biggar RJ, et al. Determinants of retrovirus (HTLV-III) antibody and immunodeficiency conditions in homosexual men. Lancet 2:711, 1984.

14. Goedert JJ, Blattner WA. The epidemiology of AIDS and related conditions. In *AIDS: Etiology Diagnosis, Treatment, and Prevention*. DeVita VT, Hellman S, Rosenberg SA (eds). J. B. Lippincott Company, New York, p. 1-30, 1985.

15. Melbye M, Biggar RJ, Ebbesen P, et al. Seroepidemiology of HTLV-III antibody in Danish homosexual men: Prevalence, transmission and disease outcome. Br Med J 289:573, 1984.

16. Mathur-Wagh U, Mildvan D, Tancovitz SR, et al. Persistent generalized lymphadenopathy in homosexual men: A 40 month follow-up and results of serology measured by Ig G ELISA (abst). International Conference on Acquired Immunodeficiency Syndrome (AIDS), Atlanta, GA, April 14-17, 1985, p. 83.

17. Groopman JE, Mayer KH, Sarngadharan MG. Seroepidemiology of human T-lymphotropic virus type III among homosexual men with the acquired immuno-

deficiency syndrome or generalized lymphadenopathy and amount asymptomatic controls in Boston. Ann Intern Med 102:334, 1985.

18. Eyster ME, Goedert JJ, Sarngadharan, MG, et al. Development and early natural history of HTLV-III antibodies in persons with hemophilia, JAMA 253:2219, 1985.

19. Fauci A. Acquired immunodeficiency syndrome (AIDS)–an update. American Gastroenterological Association Meeting, New York, May 13, 1985.

20. Testimony before the Subcommittee on Health and the Environ ment; Committee on Energy and Commerce. U.S. House of Representatives, Washington, D.C., July 22, 1985.

21. CDC. Antibodies to a retrovirus etiologically associated with acquired immunodeficiency syndrome (AIDS) in populations with increased incidence of the syndrome. Morbid Mortal Weekly Rep 33:377, 1984.

22. Landesman SH, Ginzburg HM, Weiss SH. The AIDS epidemic, N Engl J Med 312:521, 1985.

23. Fischinger PJ, Bolognesi DP. Prospects for diagnostic tests, intervention, and vaccine development in AIDS. In *AIDS: Etiology, Diagnosis, Treatment, and Prevention.* DeVita VT, Hellman S, Rosenberg SA (eds). J.B. Lippincott Company, New York, p. 55-88, 1985.

24. Spira TJ, DesJarlais DC, Marmar M, et al. Prevalence of antibody to lymphadenopathy-associated virus among drug-detoxification patients in New York (letter), N Engl J Med 311:467, 1984.

25. Review of the Public Health Services Response to AIDS. Washington, D.C. U.S. Congress Office of Technology Assessment. February 1985, p. 26.

26. Clumek N, Sonnet J, Tallman H, et al. Acquired immunodeficiency syndrome in African patients. N Engl J Med 310:492, 1984.

27. Van De Perre P, Lepage P, Kestelyn P, et al. Acquired immunodeficiency syndrome in Rwanda, Lancet 2:62, 1984.

28. Van DePerre P, Carael M, Marjorie Robert-Guroff, et

al. Female prostitutes: A risk group for infection with human T-cell lymphotropic virus type III, Lancet 2:524, 1985.

29. Biggar RJ, Johnson B, Gigase P, et al. Seropedemiology of HTLV-III in Eastern Zaire and Kenya (abst), International Conference on Acquired Immunodeficiency Syndrome, Atlanta, GA, April 14-17, 1985, p. 68.

30. Potterat JJ, Rothenberg R, Bross DC. Gonorrhea in street prostitutes. Sex Transm Dis 6:58, 1979.

31. Quinn TC. Perspectives on the future of AIDS. JAMA 253:247, 1985.

32. Bross DC. Legal aspects of STD control. In *Sexually Transmitted Diseases*. Holmes KK, Mardl P, Sparling PF, Wiesner PJ (eds). McGraw-Hill Book Company, New York, p 925-930, 1984.

33. Schultz S, Friedman S, Kistal A, et al. Declining rates of rectal and pharyngeal gonorrhea among males–New York City. Morbid Mortal Weekly Rep. 33:295, 1984.

34. Pickering J, Wiley JA, Padian, et al. Modeling acquired immunodeficiency syndrome in New York, San Francisco and Los Angeles (abst). International Conference on Acquired Immunodeficiency Syndrome, Atlanta, Ga, April 14-17, 1985, p. 37.

8

The Medical Horizon

A tremendous amount has been learned in a few short years, but it is realistic to say that our knowledge of the AIDS virus is dwarfed by what we do not know. The purpose of this section is to provide an overview of current medical understanding and delineate the medical challenges that lie ahead.

Defining the Natural History of the Disease

In its attempt to understand a disease, science endeavors to establish a "natural history" using all the means at its disposal. This term refers to the progression of a disease from beginning to conclusion, including the entire constellation of possible outcomes. In this context, "history" refers to lifetime projections of mortality (death) and morbidity (serious but not fatal conditions). "Natural" denotes the progression of an illness without medical intervention. In this context, medical science searches for ways to disrupt the natural progression of a disease in order to moderate or alter its outcome.

A simple illustration is the natural history of a patient with leukemia. Before any sort of medical interventions were developed, leukemia progressed naturally (without intervention) to its inevitably terminal conclusion. Now certain medical interventions, notably chemotherapy, can moderate the course of the disease. The natural history of leukemia is a complete description of its progression from onset to termination. It includes all of the possible routes of progression. One might say that the natural history is a synopsis of the sum total of the case histories of people affected by a disease, uninterrupted by medical intervention.

Information about the natural history of animal retroviruses suggests that the AIDS virus will remain in infected individuals indefinitely, but our information on this expected "lifetime infection" is the product of only 5 years of tracking the disease. What does the picture look like at 10 years? Fifteen? Twenty to 25 years? It appears that 5–20% of an infected population will develop AIDS within 5 years. What additional percentage will convert in years 6 to 10? Eleven to 20? Twenty to 30?

Less than 200,000 Americans were infected by the end of 1982. Most belonged to one of three high-risk groups: male homosexuals, IV drug users, or recent Haitian immigrants. Only a small percentage of these infected individuals will be identified by the end of 1985. Medical science is trying to determine the natural history of AIDS virus infection from a small unrepresentative sample of the population, infected usually for less than five years.

Early research on the natural history of the disease has been hampered by current policies that discourage symptomless individuals from having their blood tested for the AIDS virus. The "story" of the natural history of the AIDS virus will unfold as time progresses. However, the pool of infected individuals from which to glean this knowledge continues to grow at a prodigious rate, and the million or more currently infected individuals will no doubt yield a very detailed natural history of the AIDS virus (from years zero to five) by the start of the 1990s. The knowledge will be achieved at a very great cost: 100,000 or more AIDS cases and an additional 250,000 ARC cases.

It is of pressing current interest whether infection by the AIDS virus causes a predictable early set of signs or symptoms. This is referred to as the "acute phase" of the illness. Is there an initial illness that predictably takes place relatively soon after infection?

Lancet, a British medical journal, detailed a case of a nurse who accidentally pricked herself with the needle of an AIDS patient.[1] This example was made striking by the fact that the nurse actually injected a small amount of blood from a drawn syringe through the needle into her bloodstream.

The nurse reported a severe "flulike" illness which appeared 13 days after the needle prick. It was characterized by headache, mild sore throat, muscle aches, and facial pains. On the 17th day a rash appeared on her chest and trunk. The rash lasted for one week, during which time it spread to the neck and face. Fever, general depression, and swollen glands also characterized the reaction. These signs and symptoms receded and disappeared within one month of the needle stick accident.

Lancet also published a report from an Australian group evaluating homosexual men in Sydney.[2] Conversion from a negative to a positive AIDS virus blood test was documented in 12 subjects. Eleven experienced an acute mononucleosislike illness, developing a positive blood test in periods ranging from two to eight weeks. The illness was of sudden onset, lasted from 3 to 14 days, and was associated with fever, fatigue, sweats, loss of appetite, nausea, muscle aches, joint pains, headache, sore throat, diarrhea, swollen glands, and a red rash.

These cases are currently the best available documentation on the "acute phase" of AIDS virus infection. It is possible that this type of reaction is a standard part of the natural history of infection. If so, it should be possible to identify some portion of infected individuals relatively soon after infection.

Three recognized states follow the acute phase of AIDS virus infection: symptomless carrier, ARC, and full-blown AIDS. Medical investigators are actively debating whether the variety of outcomes observed so far represent *distinct end points* in a spectrum of disease (Figure 8-1) or merely various stages along a continuum inevitably leading to the *same end point* (Figure 8-2).

Figure 8-1 illustrates the prevailing five-year model (Model A). Following acute AIDS virus infection, patients generally remain symptomless for at least one year. These individuals usually harbor live, transmittable AIDS virus and are properly considered potentially infectious carriers. Although some of the symptomless patients may not be shedding virus and are unlikely to be infectious, current technology does not allow us to identify and segregate these individuals into a separate group. Some patients progress from the carrier state to ARC. Others seem to progress from the symptomless state to full-blown AIDS. Some ARC patients develop AIDS.

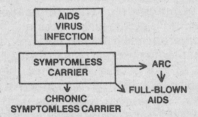

Figure 8-1. Model A illustrates the current observed pattern. AIDS virus infection seems to produce three possible outcomes—symptomless carriers, ARC and AIDS. Some individuals progress from the symptomless carrier state to ARC. Others seem to progress directly from the symptomless carrier state to full-blown AIDS. Some ARC patients develop AIDS.

Figure 8-2 depicts an alternative model (Model B). Advocates believe that the currently defined clinical states are different antecedents to the same conclusion. Over time the AIDS virus will inevitably weaken and destroy the immune systems of infected individuals, rendering them progressively more susceptible to ARC and full-blown AIDS. Proponents of Model B agree the "end" states illustrated in Figure 8-1 are a misleading representation of the natural history of AIDS virus infection based on only five years of empiric observation. In contrast, supporters of Model A note many ARC patients have lymphadenopathy syndrome, which seems to remain medically stable for several years, with the immune system seeming to be damaged but not getting any worse.

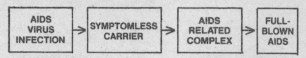

Figure 8-2. Model B suggests that the virus will not only remain inside infected individuals indefinitely, but that periods of active replication and destruction of the immune system are inevitable.

Some investigators are advocating a modification of Model B, because a variety of disorders are appearing in individuals infected by the AIDS virus that are potentially fatal or seriously debilitating but are not necessarily associated with the immune impairment observed in either ARC or full-blown AIDS. These complications of AIDS virus infection are included in another group referred to as AIDS virus–related disorders, or AVRDS. Model C shows this proposed natural history of AIDS virus infection in Figure 8-3.

One case illustrating AVRDS occurred in an infected medical school teacher. This professor developed dementia without any usual manifestations of ARC or full-blown AIDS. Careful evaluation suggested the professor's senility resulted from AIDS virus replication within his central nervous system. No other explanation was found, and AIDS virus grew from samples of brain tissue and cerebrospinal fluid.

Other AVRDS include cases of children born without brains or with half brains. The mothers were infected with AIDS virus, and autopsies of the infants revealed AIDS virus in neurological tissue. A strange form of pancreatic cancer has occurred in young infected individuals. Patients with AIDS virus infection are more likely to develop lymphoma or Hodgkin's disease. Whether the AIDS virus causes or facilitates the development of these blood malignancies has not been determined.

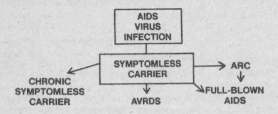

Figure 8-3. Model C expands on Model A by including a group for AIDS Virus Related Disorders (AVRDS). The current CDC surveillance definition of AIDS does not have a separate category for AVRDS and includes other (i.e. not specifically associated with immune system damage) life-threatening complications such as lymphoma in the full-blown AIDS group. (See Appendix B and C.)

More information and time will help clarify the relationship between AIDS virus and associated medical conditions. Although the model that best depicts the natural course of AIDS virus infection is uncertain, it appears clear that infected individuals face very serious long-term medical consequences.

With respect to the five-year mortality (cumulative death rate), recent figures roughly suggest 10% of an infected population will develop full-blown AIDS within three years of infection and 80% of those diagnosed with full-blown AIDS die within three years of the diagnosis. Therefore, it appears that AIDS virus causes an 8% cumulative mortality rate over the first six years of infection. This translates into a 1.3% annual death rate.

Since infected individuals are probably contagious within weeks of exposure, the AIDS virus creates almost immediate, universal morbidity (associated complications). So rather than ask who experiences complications from AIDS virus infection, the real issues are what complications and when. The best estimates indicate between 30–45% of a population will develop full-blown AIDS or ARC within 5 years of transmission. The percentage of patients that will present with AVRDS is unknown. The 5-year morbidity of AIDS virus infection is bad; apparently all infected individuals will suffer significant medical consequences. Even more distressing, the outlook for 10 years, 20 years, 30 years, and beyond is likely to be worse, possibly much worse.

Directly related to the morbidity and mortality of AIDS virus infection are questions about cofactors. Because the natural history at five years appears quite variable from individual to individual, some investigators postulate an important role for cofactors. In this context, cofactors are independent influences that may affect the outcome of AIDS virus infection. Cofactors may trigger or enhance AIDS virus replication, further damaging the host's immune system. Current research is focusing on many factors including natural aging; germs such as cytomegalovirus, papillomavirus, Epstein-Barr virus, herpes virus, hepatitis B virus, and HTLV-I; underlying diseases such as diabetes and cancer; smoking, alcohol, and recreational drug use; and psychosocial influences such as life stress, exhaustion, depression, and anxiety.

The idea that cofactors are necessary to trigger the active phase of viral replication has not been borne out in research.[3] The existence of previously healthy symptomless carriers who suddenly, without explanation, experience replicative attacks on their T-helper cells also argues that cofactors may be *facilitative* but are not *necessary* for replication.

Dr. Gallo believes long-term antigenic stimulation may be an important cofactor.[4] An antigen is a substance, foreign to the body, that stimulates the production of antibodies by the immune system. Antigens include foreign proteins, bacteria, viruses, pollen, and other materials. In order to produce an antibody response to an antigen, the immune system must activate T-cells and B-cells. Stimulation to the T-cells may shake the AIDS virus from dormancy. The virus emerges from the T-helper cell's genes and begins to rapidly replicate. Millions of new AIDS viruses freely circulate throughout the host's body fluids looking for new cells to infect.

Immune system activation creates double trouble. Not only are previously dormant viruses stimulated to replicate but also activated T-helper cells appear to be more susceptible to deadly AIDS virus attack. This cycle is vicious—more stimulation leads to greater activation, which creates both more virus and cells more vulnerable to infection. Indeed, the AIDS virus itself may produce chronic antigenic stimulation, resulting in accelerated immune system destruction.

Many viruses produce chronic antigen stimulation, and some viruses appear to influence the outcome of AIDS virus infection in a predictable way. For instance, B-cell lymphoma often attacks individuals concurrently infected with both Epstein-Barr and AIDS viruses. Laboratory evidence suggests immune system activation by the Epstein-Barr virus makes B-cells vulnerable to AIDS virus attack. AIDS virus incorporation into the genes of B-cells may lead directly or indirectly to the development of lymphoma.

Investigators wonder what cofactor or cofactors account for the occurrence of Kaposi's sarcoma in 40–50% of homosexual patients with full-blown AIDS. By comparison, only about 4% of all heterosexual intravenous drug users with AIDS and about 12% of Haitian AIDS patients develop Kaposi's sarcoma. Dr. Gallo speculates[4] the difference may be the papillomavirus, which causes venereal warts and is endemic in homosexual communities. Interestingly, several researchers have reported patients with Kaposi's without any apparent immune abnormality from the AIDS virus.[4]

Unfortunately, the genetic mechanisms that link different viral cofactors and AIDS virus to specific outcomes are unknown. The actual importance of coinfection to the natural history of AIDS virus infection is a modern medical mystery. Among the theoretical cofactors being considered that might influence the outcome of AIDS virus infection, long-term antigenic stimulation and, in particular, concurrent viral infection are receiving considerable research attention.

Environmental conditions are often mentioned as possible cofactors in the development of AIDS, including malnutrition, poor sanitation, and poor overall health habits. These conditions are present in many of the AIDS cases reported out of Africa, suggesting that these factors create a fertile environment in which AIDS virus can easily attack and replicate.

When the role of cofactors in the onset of AIDS is defined, more accurate long-range morbidity and mortality projections will be available. The idea that the AIDS virus can be triggered out of dormancy by another illness or medical trauma (such as a heart attack) is troublesome news for infected individuals. It is possible, for example, that Rock Hudson's 1981 heart bypass operation triggered the AIDS virus into replication. It is possible that AIDS virus carriers are never past a "danger point" and will always have to live with the fear of a sudden attack on their immune system.

To summarize, the description of the natural history of the AIDS virus is one major challenge on the medical horizon. At present there exists a vague picture of the effects of the virus in small subsets of populations over a 3- to 5-year period. Because the virus is so persistent and so many young people are infected, the 10-, 20-, 30-, and even 50-year picture is important. Even in a subject as basic as defining the nature of the disease, the magnitude of the questions yet to be answered dwarfs current understanding.

Understanding Transmission of the Virus

The means by which the AIDS virus may be generally spread have been delineated. The virus can be transmitted sexually, through infected blood and blood products, through the sharing of contaminated needles, and from mother to child. While there are unanswered questions about each of these methods, sexual transmission clearly represents the greatest threat to the largest number of people.

The AIDS virus has been cultured from the blood, tears, saliva, semen, and urine of infected individuals.[5-7] Therefore, the Food and Drug Administration recommends refraining from any sexual practice that involves their exchange. It is likely, however, that certain sexual practices are more facilitative for the transmission of the virus than others.

In the first reports of AIDS, receptive anal intercourse was the sexual activity that correlated most strongly with its development. This type of sex is believed to be facilitative of the transmission of the AIDS virus for two reasons. The first is that the virus has a high concentration in semen.[8] The second is that the rectal lining is easily damaged.[9] This combination of a potential portal to the bloodstream being flooded with a concentrated source of the virus creates a viable transmission opportunity.

It has been suggested that the AIDS virus *must* have a portal to the bloodstream in order for transmission to take place. Clearly this can happen in forms of sexuality other than anal intercourse. In vigorous vaginal intercourse the lining can be damaged, creating a portal to the bloodstream. It is simply unknown if there *must* be a portal to the bloodstream in order for sexual transmission of the AIDS virus to occur. An Australian report published in *Lancet* September 1985 provides indirect but very relevant information on this subject.[10] Eight women were artificially inseminated with semen from a symptomless carrier of the AIDS virus. The exposure was limited to previously frozen semen, gently placed in the vagina. Four of these eight women were infected, although there was no evidence for a direct portal to the bloodstream.

Because the AIDS virus has been cultured from the

saliva of infected individuals, the FDA currently recommends that infected individuals refrain from "French" kissing. This is a reasonable precaution. Dr. Zaki Salahuddin has provided an example in which intimate kissing was the only possible vector of transmission: an elderly infected woman whose only exposure was kissing her AIDS husband, an impotent transfusion recipient.[11] All other documented examples of sexual transmission have involved other forms of sexual activity. The idea of running a controlled experiment limited to intimate kissing between an infected and uninfected individual is ethically tenuous. So, for the foreseeable future intimate kissing will continue to be identified as a dangerous activity.

In spite of the above recommendation, epidemiological studies of AIDS virus transmission suggest oral-oral and oral-genital contact are not as risky as penile-vaginal and penile-rectal contact. It seems stomach acid can typically destroy the AIDS virus before it finds a portal to the bloodstream. The stomach's protective role may be compromised if infected bodily secretions first reach a canker sore, oral ulceration, fever blister, cut lip, or injured gum. Many Americans do not have stomach acid due to a variety of reasons, including ulcer surgery, natural aging, or some medications. These Americans may have increased susceptibility to AIDS virus infection from oral-oral and oral-genital contact.

Some medical investigators believe background antigenic stimulation plays a significant role in the successful transmission of AIDS virus. They postulate an individual is more likely to be infected by the AIDS virus if his or her immune system is actively producing antibodies at the time of exposure to the AIDS contagion. Immune system stimulation appears to accelerate viral replication and T-cell infection and death. Ironically, perhaps from the moment the AIDS virus finds a cellular beachhead in a host with an active immune system, the attack dramatically amplifies.

The first case of AIDS transmission through heterosexual contact appeared in late 1982,[12] although AIDS cases in heterosexual intravenous drug users appeared a year earlier. By the end of 1985, this type of case had appeared in 36 states. Heterosexual spread has also been well documented in Africa, Germany, France, and Haiti. It is established that prostitution accounts for a large part of heterosexual spread in Africa, Germany, and Haiti, and the same is postulated for the United States. In the history of the disease to date, there has been a tendency on the part of the CDC to slot American heterosexual AIDS cases into "acceptable" risk groups, especially intravenous drug users, which has seemingly drawn attention away from the problem. (See Chapter 7.)

In Japan, where the disease AIDS is rare, a study of HTLV-I provides an interesting perspective on female-to-male transmission. In married couples where the "conductor" was male, the spouse was a carrier of the virus in almost every case, while less than half the husbands of infected women were themselves carriers of HTLV-I.[13] Such findings inspired comparison with a study of HTLV-carrying Japanese monkeys, in which carrier males regularly transmitted the virus to females in mating, while no male had been found contaminated despite the added probability of exposure due to the males' being polygamous.[13] This has been attributed to the HTLV's being a "parasite," present only in host cells and chiefly in T-lymphocytes, which abound in both simian and human sperm. Contagion appears to result from the introduction of infected cells to receptive mucous membranes. Although HTLV-I and HTLV-III (AIDS virus) are in the same family, caution must be observed in applying these studies directly to AIDS, since the germs, though related, are distinct and different viruses. Dr. Gallo cautions that the AIDS virus replicates far more rapidly and is far more contagious than HTLV-I.

Comparison of the AIDS virus with herpes simplex II (genital herpes) is also interesting, though less fruitful. People infected with the herpes virus are not always infectious. The herpes virus remains dormant for a great deal of the time. Only during periods of "shedding" can it be transmitted. Shedding generally creates visible signs such as blisters on the genitals or the mouth. Infected individuals can choose to abstain from sexual activity during these periods and therefore reduce appreciably the risk of infecting a sexual partner.

It is possible that the AIDS virus follows a similar pattern and that infected individuals are infectious only during certain periods. If this is so, it is likely that sexual activity during noninfectious periods would be safe. The hope that this possibility represents should be tempered by the reality that the AIDS virus does not create noticeable signs or symptoms a great deal of the time. It is possible that although infected individuals are not always infectious it will be difficult or impossible to determine when these safe times exist.

The sharing of contaminated needles by intravenous drug users seems to be an efficient way to transmit the virus. It is estimated that two-thirds or more of the New York City IV drug users are infected. On the other hand, a number of "needle pricks" of contaminated needles by · health care workers has been reported with only one case of transmission taking place. The example of the British nurse was unique because a small amount of infected blood was actually injected into her bloodstream. This suggests with respect to infected blood (and presumably other body fluids) a "critical mass" of contagion must be injected.

The period of "dormancy" (between infection and the appearance of signs or symptoms of AIDS or ARC—also called "incubation") has been frequently discussed. Less attention has been given to the apparent period of "latency" (between infection and the production of measurable antibodies). In humans, this latent period is generally believed to be from two to eight weeks but has been measured to be longer than six months.[11] In other words, over a six-month period has elapsed between infection and a positive reading on the AIDS virus blood test. In two studies, chimpanzees did not develop measurable antibodies until three months after exposure.[14,15]

This latent period has obvious implications for transmission of the AIDS virus via donated blood or blood products. What is the precise mechanism by which the AIDS virus is transmitted through infected blood? What causes the variability in this latency period? Is it related to the transmitter or receiver? These sorts of issues will be on researchers' minds as they wait to see if the screening procedures that have been put in place will eliminate transfusion-associated transmission of the AIDS virus. Because of the long (two- to five-year) incubation period for transfusion-related AIDS, the efficacy of blood screening will not be fully known in this decade.

Transmission of the AIDS virus from mother to infant or unborn child has been observed. It is apparent that the virus can be transmitted directly, through the placenta, or indirectly, through infected milk. In one study 16 mothers infected with virus (15 initially were symptomless) gave birth to infants who were infected with the virus. However, 5 of these women subsequently gave birth to infants who were not infected with the AIDS virus.[16]

It is clear that mothers can infect infants with the AIDS virus. For this reason pregnancy should be avoided by couples in which there is an AIDS virus infection. On the other hand, it is apparent that not all infected mothers will bear infected children. What are the factors controlling transplacental and perinatal transmission?

At present an average of two children per day are born in New York City to women who are infected with the AIDS virus. Approximately half of the children have the virus. A very puzzling anecdote involves *twins* born to an infected mother. One infant was infected at birth and the other was not.[4] In the future will it be possible to define a set of safeguards by which parents infected with the AIDS virus may safely conceive children?

These findings underline the whole question of natural

immunity and natural susceptibility. Are some people more susceptible to infection with the AIDS virus? Are some people less susceptible to infection with the AIDS virus? If so, why? What can be learned from this sort of natural immunity that can help slow the spread of the virus? Blood collected in 1972 on healthy Ugandan children showed a 67% rate of AIDS virus infection.[17] This is intriguing, as it may indicate either an adapted immunity or perhaps infection with a less virulent strain of AIDS virus. Suffice it to say that no evidence of any sort of human immunity has reliably presented itself as yet, and that findings of this sort are probably remote on the scientific horizon.

The final issue to be explored related to transmission is the possibility of nonhuman vectors. A vector (usually a biting insect) is a carrier which transfers an infective agent from one host to another. A vector in whose body the infecting germ develops or multiplies before becoming infective to the recipient individual is called a biological vector. A vector that transmits an infective germ from one host to another but which is not essential to the life cycle of the agent is known as a mechanical vector. An insect vector can be either the primary mode of transmission or can simply add to a more typical pattern of spread.

Dr. Carl Saxinger, a collaborator of Dr. Gallo at the NCI, is currently investigating the epidemiology of HTLV-I.[4] Unlike the AIDS virus, HTLV-I has been endemic in human populations for centuries. Dr. Saxinger has discovered that 20% of the normal adult population of Papua, New Guinea, has evidence of HTLV-I infection. This retrovirus was probably introduced into the native population of New Guinea by Japanese soldiers during World War II, and spread rapidly throughout the population. Dr. Saxinger speculates insect-borne transmission may have contributed to this dramatic growth in prevalence. Although Dr. Gallo warns not to overinterpret this epidemiological data, he cautions that if HTLV-I can be spread by insects, it is likely so can AIDS virus.

There is epidemiological evidence both in America and in Africa that mosquitoes have the potential to transmit the virus. There is a clustering of infection in the small, impoverished agricultural community of Belle Glade, Florida. There were 37 AIDS cases reported in Belle Glade, a town of only 17,000 residents, by early 1985. Significantly, more than half did not fit into any of the standardized "high risk" categories. The prevalence of mosquitoes in combination with a great deal of unexplained infection suggests that mosquitoes may transmit the AIDS virus.

Many researchers acknowledge mosquitoes can theoretically serve as a mechanical vector for the AIDS virus. The insect can transmit the virus by first biting an infected individual and then an uninfected individual. The mosquito, when it first bites, injects a natural anesthetic substance. This material may be contaminated with AIDS contagion picked up from the previous blood meal.

Dr. Peter Drotman of the CDC believes if this were a common pattern of transmission, we would be seeing additional cases in individuals who share an environment with infected persons.[18] In spite of extensive surveillance efforts in this country, such evidence is generally lacking (Belle Glade being the notable exception).

Malaria and yellow fever are diseases that depend on mosquitoes as a biological vector. Epidemiological control of these requires insect eradication and possibly vaccination. At present, most investigators do not believe insects are a biological vector for the AIDS virus. However, there are extremely worrisome theoretical possibilities. Some speculate that the AIDS virus may evolve to a point where it can genetically incorporate itself into an established insect-borne virus or parasite, potentially facilitating transmission.[19] Others suggest the AIDS virus may produce a variant strain that may have an insect-borne phase to its life cycle. Although insect-borne transmission of the AIDS virus now seems only to be a theoretical problem, epidemiologists will continue aggressively looking for evidence of insect-borne spread.

Further knowledge about transmission, particularly sexual transmission, is difficult to come by. Controlled human laboratory studies are ethically untenable. Animal models may have limited applicability. The period of latency (between infection and the production of measurable antibodies) adds to the problems in isolating specific sexual activity as facilitative for transmission.

One promising available tool is to interview infected individuals extensively and draw some inferences about sexual habits that seem to facilitate transmission. Such study of homosexual men indicated that transmission strongly correlated with number of sexual partners and receptive anal intercourse.

This kind of epidemiological study to investigate the suspected cases of American heterosexual transmission represents an important avenue for research. Interviews of this nature are delicate and their use is controversial. As such, this research tool may continue to be underutilized until large numbers of heterosexual AIDS cases develop.

The challenges to medical science to define the conditions under which the AIDS virus can and cannot be transmitted are considerable, if not insurmountable. Currently available medical technology cannot absolutely detect the presence of the virus in infected individuals. The lay person has no means with which to identify (or even suggest) the presence of infection. The more medical science understands about the nature of the AIDS virus, the more vexing the problems related to slowing its infectious spread appear to be.

An Overview of Potential Interventions

There are three basic ways to moderate the effects of an infectious disease: prevent the spread, develop a vaccine, and develop an effective program of treatment.

Preventing the Spread

Because of the uncertainties related to the prognosis of AIDS-virus-positive people, it is clear that one current urgent need is to prevent the spread of the virus. One obvious step that can be taken is to embark on a widespread program of "risk reduction education." Campaigns to reduce casual, anonymous sex have been implemented in a number of gay communities.

A study of 500 homosexual and bisexual men showed that 90% had reduced the frequency of "unsafe" sexual practices.[20] Two-thirds reported that they were either celibate, monogamous, or practicing safe sex as a result of the AIDS epidemic. The degree to which changes such as these are due to risk reduction education or simply fear of the disease itself is not known. This ambiguity should not, however, be interpreted as a reason to delay in the implementation of such programs.

The greatest obstacles to such a program in heterosexual America are lack of willpower and unwillingness to take the threat seriously. It is unfortunate that many gay communities became aware of the dangers of sexual promiscuity too late to prevent the epidemic spread of the virus. In New York and San Francisco it is estimated that 70–90% of the sexually active homosexual men are infected. The question of whether promiscuous heterosexual America will follow a similar pattern, only "sobering up" after larger percentages are infected, remains to be seen.

Developing a Vaccine

The idea of developing a vaccine for the AIDS virus strikes many at first thought as a promising avenue. However, there are a number of theoretical and logistical considerations which indicate that the development of an effective vaccine is a number of years in the future.

When the announcement was made that the cause of AIDS had been determined, many people presumed that a vaccination would be developed in a fairly short period of time. Since the turn of the century, vaccines have effectively eliminated smallpox, diphtheria, and polio as public health concerns.

There are a number of characteristics of the AIDS virus that make the development of an effective vaccine difficult and perhaps impossible. One issue yet to be resolved is how mny different variations of AIDS virus exist. Dr. Robert Gallo at the National Cancer Institute has already examined 18 different AIDS virus isolates.[21] The AIDS virus is referred to as HTLV-III in the United States, LAV in France, and ARV in other parts of the world. The AIDS epidemic has a different pattern in Africa than in the West. The virus itself also appears to vary geographically. There is evidence to suggest that even within a single geographical location, there may be more than one variant of the AIDS virus.

There has also been a correlation that seems to hold between number of sexual partners and the development of AIDS. It is possible that this is due solely to the increased risk of initial infection as a result of promiscuity, as sexually active people in any population with some degree of infectivity run a greater risk for infection than those who are less sexually active. But another hypothesis is that a variety of variants of the AIDS virus exist and that multiple infection with variants of the virus is an important cofactor for converting from infection to AIDS. This hypothesis suggests that people who have been infected with one variant of the AIDS virus can reduce their risk of developing AIDS by regulating their sexual activity. By avoiding exposure to another variant of the AIDS virus, they are reducing the possibility of triggering the active phase of replication.

This type of speculation underscores the prospect that if a number of variants of the virus exist, a number of vaccinations may need to be developed to protect against this. The closest animal virus to the AIDS virus is *Visna* virus, another retrovirus causing progressive encephalitis (brain inflammation) in sheep. Multiple variations of the same virus have been found in a single infected animal.[22] If this holds true for the AIDS virus in humans, it would significantly compound the problems in formulating an effective vaccine preparation.

A variation on the "multiple variants" theory is the possibility that the virus might change subtly but perceptibly over time. Thus a vaccine would be effective only for a period of time. This is true of annual flu vaccines. If this is the case, the long incubation period for AIDS or ARC adds to the possible pitfall of developing vaccines for "yesterday's" virus. Dr. Haseltine of Harvard says, "Trying to develop a vaccine for AIDS is like trying to hit a moving target."

No effective vaccine is commercially available for *any* germ of the retrovirus family, of which the AIDS virus is a member.[22] A vaccine has been developed for the feline leukemia virus. However, there is considerable controversy in the veterinarian community as to whether or not this vaccine is safe.

Research to develop a vaccine for the AIDS virus is an international priority. Initial work in America is being conducted at the National Cancer Institute's Frederick Cancer Research Facility in Frederick, Maryland. A vaccine is essentially an injection of either modified avirulent virus, inactivated virus, or viral subunits which stimulate the recipient's immune system to produce virus-neutralizing antibodies. Thus far research efforts have yet to identify antibodies capable of neutralizing the AIDS virus. Until this hurdle is cleared the development of an effective vaccine is clearly impossible.

Keep in mind that it took 11 years of concentrated research to develop an effective vaccine for hepatitis B. And the AIDS problem is even more complex, involving elimination of a virus that incorporates itself into the genetic material of the host, and thus presents conceptual and experimental challenges never before faced in microbiology. The situation would seem hopeless were it not for some recent technological developments that at least offer avenues of exploration. Currently a number of new biotechnical advances in recombinant DNA techniques and genetic probes are proving useful.

Having achieved production of a vaccine, the process of clinical trials will be similarly formidable. The illness' periods of dormancy (time between infection and clinical manifestations) and latency (time between exposure and development of measurable antibodies) pose logistical problems in identifying high-risk but uninfected subjects. The same problems may recur in identifying their time (not to mention means) of infection. Finally, the virus's potential for reactivation at any time will require prolonged observation of test subjects.

Dr. James Curran of the Centers for Disease Control is one of the most moderate voices authoritative about AIDS. His counsel often emphasizes progress and the positive possibilities inherent in the present situation. Even Dr. Curran admits that by the time a vaccine might be developed it will be necessary to vaccinate all individuals before they become sexually active. For Dr. Curran to make that admission is more significant than might be initially imagined. The message is clear. For the foreseeable future a workable vaccine is a bad bet and the only truly effective intervention for the prevention of the spread of the virus remains responsible sexual behavior.

Developing an Effective Program of Treatment

There are a variety of therapeutic procedures to combat some of the various clinical manifestations of AIDS and ARC patients. AIDS patients with Kaposi's sarcoma are treated with systemic chemotherapy. However, there are no data to show that treatment improves survival, so currently available chemotherapy at best is palliative. In spite of some temporary benefit on the existing tumors, no current chemotherapeutic regimen for treating Kaposi's sarcoma has been found to prevent the appearance of new lesions or to consistently improve the underlying immune deficiency.

Medical investigators believe the ideal treatment may require a combination of immunotherapy and chemotherapy.

Pneumocystis carinii pneumonia is the most common form of pneumonia in patients with AIDS. Most patients with AIDS will develop *Pneumocystis carinii* infection during their illness. The initial symptoms are nonspecific and include cough, fever, chills, and shortness of breath. It takes an average of 28 days from the onset of symptoms until *Pneumocystis carinii* is usually documented in AIDS patients.[23] Once the pneumonia has been diagnosed, there are several antibiotics (specifically trimethopri-sulfamethoxazole or pentamidine) that are useful. About 60–70% of AIDS patients with *Pneumocystis* pneumonia when treated with antibiotics will survive this life-threatening crisis. However, recurrences are common. In children with leukemia, trimethopri-sulfamethoxazole administered daily as prophylaxis does reduce the incidence of *Pneumocystis* pneumonia. However, there are no studies to show that similar benefit and allergic reactions are common in patients with AIDS.

AIDS patients are susceptible to more than 30 germs that can become life threatening due to the damaged immune system. Many of these germs were previously seen infecting only cancer-chemotherapy and organ-transplant patients. These conditions are treated according to individual requirements with standard therapies. AIDS patients can exhibit many other problems, including mental deterioration, swollen glands, fever, unintentional weight loss, diarrhea, and night sweats.

Standard therapeutic procedures for treating the various clinical manifestations of AIDS and ARC patients do not solve the underlying problem—a damaged immune system. Research has in some cases developed drugs that by necessity are a great deal more potent than the agents normally used. This increased potency is needed to overcome the effect of immune deficiency. Although some of these new agents show promise in moderating specific clinical problems observed in AIDS patients, they do not represent great hope even for patients whose ailments they counteract. Typically, an infection will recur or another equally life-threatening infection will take place.

A significant medical hurdle is the need to develop a drug that crosses the "blood-brain barrier." Recent evidence discloses that the AIDS virus can penetrate the brain and cause central nervous system damage. An effective drug, therefore, will need to cross into the central nervous system and protect the brain from infection. Prolonged treatment and observation of patients will be necessary due to the virus's potential for reactivation at a later time. As in vaccine research, the path is fraught with conceptual barriers and long proving times, and it will be years before any treatment clears the FDA's rigorous requirements and is put to general use.

Clinical Trials

It is important to note that the Food and Drug Administration (FDA) must approve every new medical therapy, and that the process of gaining FDA approval is slow and tedious. Typically, there is a long stage of animal tests and safety trials before clinical trials in humans are allowed. A drug must demonstrate both safety and effectiveness to receive FDA approval for manufacture and sale.

Once a drug is thought to be a potentially effective agent in some disease, it must prove its worth in an elaborate set of procedures called "clinical trials." These procedures are quite conservative, and the requirements to pass to the next step are strict. For example, data obtained in another country are generally not permitted to support an argument for a drug to be used in this country. As a result, studies that were performed with methodological rigor abroad have been repeated in America to satisfy this requirement. This takes both money and time.

Antiviral agents are being investigated as possible AIDS treatments. Antiviral agents attempt to halt the replication of the virus once it has infected the bloodstream. Here are some of the procedures that would have to be adhered to by an investigator attempting to prove the worth of a particular antiviral agent:

The first step is to culture the virus in a test tube and introduce the agent. The agent's effectiveness in preventing replication of the virus in the test tube is then studied. This is referred to as *in vitro* study ("in a glass").

After the agent has been demonstrated to be effective *in vitro*, FDA approval may be granted for testing with animals. A proposal must be presented to a medical research facility which has been approved by the FDA for drug testing. The proposal must include both a theoretical explanation justifying potential benefit and *in vitro* empirical evidence of effectiveness.

This proposal is presented to an internal council of the medical center called an Institutional Review Board. A typical council is comprised of scientists, doctors, and lay advisors such as clergy. The council passes judgment on both the potential effectiveness of the agent under consideration and the ethics of the proposed animal trials.

If the drug passes approval, it is tried in animals. Due to the long incubation period, and the fact that AIDS is rarely observed naturally in animals, this phase of testing focuses on ascertaining safety, not effectiveness. Does the drug cause any side effects? What is the maximum dosage that does not produce toxic reaction? Even without attempting to prove effectiveness, this level of clinical trial takes time. The drug must show that it does not produce toxic long- or short-term effects.

If a research drug shows itself to be effective *in vitro* and safe in animals, a proposal can be written and, following FDA approval, submitted to the Institutional Review Board seeking permission to use the drug on a trial basis with a limited number of people. The proposal is presented in the form of a protocol which includes a detailed description of the research design and methodology, as well as a plan for analyzing the data collected. The protocol also includes a copy of the informed consent form which a patient must sign before entering into clinical trial. The consent form details the potential risks, as well as the hoped for benefits with the study. The purpose of the first trial with human subjects is primarily to determine the safety, not the efficacy of the research drug. Only after the drug has been shown to be reasonably safe can investigators submit proposals that specifically address the issue of effectiveness.

This is a political sore spot, since most AIDS patients see the initial human studies to determine safety as a waste of time. Because of their plight, AIDS patients are generally quite willing to volunteer for any sort of therapy that has even a chance of being effective. FDA protocols limiting experimental drug therapy to the minimum group that would satisfy statistical requirements has been severely criticized by gay-rights lobbyists.

It is quite possible that the antiviral agent will be more effective in preventing replication in symptomless carriers. This dilemma has been illustrated in the publicized example of HPA-23, an antiviral agent French scientists are using. Thanks in some part to the publicity of the Rock Hudson case, the FDA has approved its experimental use in terminally ill AIDS patients. Unfortunately, these patients have an immune system so badly damaged that the drug may not improve their condition. It may, however, be of some use if applied in the earlier stages of AIDS and ARC patients.

If an experiment on the antiviral agent were run on symptomless carriers, it would be much more difficult to analyze. Apparently a large percentage of symptomless carriers will remain symptomless for a number of years, without the introduction of an antiviral agent. It is more likely that approval would be given for testing the antiviral agent on AIDS patients, although they may be least likely to show effects. An investigator who wishes to experiment on subjects beyond this strict protocol may be able to apply for approval on what is known as a "compassionate basis."

The seriousness of the AIDS dilemma may help speed up some of the normally glacial bureaucratic delays.

An experimental design commonly used in clinical trials is double-blind placebo controlled. In this, one group is given a placebo (such as a sugar pill) and another group is given the study drug. Neither investigator nor subject knows when the actual agent will be given.

A further variation is the *crossover*, in which each subject will receive the true agent for a period of time and a placebo for a different period of time. The objective of this sort of research is to prove beyond a doubt that a drug is both safe and useful.

Since the AIDS virus apparently cannot be eliminated completely from infected individuals, it is always a threat to resume replication. That is why this stage of clinical trials is expected to take the longest for antiviral agents. The long course of AIDS means it will take a long time to prove safety and efficacy. Any agent to prevent replication may have to be used continuously over the life of the individual. This naturally slows the clinical-trials procedure for antiviral agents and draws out the question of long-range side effects, which must be satisfactorily answered before approval is given.

Closely related to the subject of clinical trials is a series of troubling ethical questions. For example, imagine an agent that is proven to reduce infectivity but has potential side effects. Should this be available to those who wish to risk the side effects? Should it be required, for example, in infected individuals who refuse to curtail their sexual activity, such as prostitutes?

There are also ethical considerations of double-blind studies involving potentially effective antiviral or immune booster agents. What are the ethics of asking some people to go without a potentially effective agent when they have AIDS? In a crossover study, what are the implications of taking someone off a treatment that seems to be working and go on a placebo? If it is clear that a subject is running the risk of life-threatening consequences, how does one justify taking them off therapy?

One medical intervention being discussed is a series of antibody shots given in a sequence shortly after infection. Hepatitis can be suppressed in this manner. In this procedure people recently exposed to hepatitis are injected with antibodies extracted from the blood of previously infected individuals. These shots generally prevent the exposed individual from developing hepatitis infection.

One of the problems in developing this kind of therapy is the risk of using infectious materials which may cause the disease you are attempting to prevent. What are the medical ethics of trying to develop this kind of intervention?

Hypothetically, it would be ideal to be able to target the infected T-helper cells early after infection and genetically "carve out" the virus before it begins to replicate. This is not within the scope of technology and likely will not be for decades to come.

There are currently six drugs close to or in clinical trials that attempt to block the replication of the AIDS virus in infected individuals. Some of the drugs attempt to block the integration of the virus into the genetic structure of the T-helper cells. Others attempt to block its reemergence from the gene. All of these drugs have shown *in vitro* effectiveness. Several have worrisome side effects. These drugs are detailed in Chapter 3, pages 77–80.

Another series of drugs is being investigated. These attempt to boost a damaged immune system. Even if the replication of the AIDS virus is blocked in AIDS patients, the immune system must be restored. A number of these agents do give a boost to the immune system, but none yet show promise of being able to restore its abilities to a state approaching normal.

Antiviral agents and immune boosters represent the best hope for the development of some sort of effective treatment. Researchers believe a successful therapeutic regimen for AIDS patients will likely be a combination of these two types of drugs.

Because of the dismal plight of patients with full-blown AIDS, the FDA may be willing to approve limited clinical trial usage of experimental therapies on a "compassionate basis." With the average life expectancy of an AIDS patient remaining at 18 months, it is understandable that those involved in trying to develop a cure will voice a degree of guarded optimism. But it is unrealistic to imagine that an effective treatment program will appear before 1990.

Conclusion: There Is Cause for Alarm

After examining some of the challenges that stand in the way of medical science with respect to the AIDS virus one can begin to appreciate the magnitude of the problem. Drs. Goedert and Blattner of the NCI recommend "a major investment in research in order to prevent an epidemic of tragic global proportions."[24]

There are a number of difficulties involved in even attempting to define the natural history and transmission pattern of the AIDS virus. There is evidence that the AIDS virus will be widely transmitted through heterosexual activity in the United States. It has been transmitted quite effectively in Africa through that means.

Since the age of antibiotics, the public has maintained a simplistic faith in the ability of researchers to root out all disease. Medical science has indeed produced miracles: the conquest of polio, smallpox, and diphtheria; the treatment of tuberculosis; and the containment of malaria. But many diseases still evade cure. Cancer is a notable example. There are signs that AIDS will continue to be as perplexing a problem as cancer.

Vaccination and treatment for AIDS may be realized in the next *few decades*. In the meantime it is absolutely imperative to moderate the spread of the virus. In the time it took to read this chapter, ten or more Americans were infected with the virus. Statistics show that one of them will die of AIDS by early 1990.

It has been suggested that this is an alarmist message. It has been suggested that people should not be frankly confronted with the truth about medical science's current frustrations in trying to develop a response to the threat represented by the AIDS virus. It has been suggested that we should wait, that we should procrastinate "until more is known" to begin painting apocalyptic visions. It is hard to understand why it is worse to "shock" people with the truth than to allow them to continue to run the risk of acquiring a potentially fatal sexually transmitted disease. Dispassionate analysis of the "state of the art" of medical science does not allow one to feel very much comfort.

Infection with the AIDS virus creates at the very least a state of permanent medical ambiguity and at the worst, disease and death. It is therefore hard to understand the delay the federal government has shown in "sounding the alarm." It seems as though prevention of "hysteria" has been a more important policy objective than the prevention of further infection. The amount of "hysteria" generated by suggesting that the virus may infect more than 10 million Americans by the end of this decade with little hope for an effective treatment program in sight should not be disregarded. But it can in no way compare to the hysteria that will take place if such a scenario actually comes to pass.

Those who would downplay the threat that AIDS represents would do well to walk the streets of the gay areas of New York and San Francisco. More than half the gay men in these cities are infected with the virus. Ask those men if they would be willing to "turn the clock back" five years. Ask those men if the short-term benefits of a liberated sensuality are worth the death, disease, and depression they now have come to live with.

Those voices who currently merchandise caution in sounding the alarm about the threat of AIDS to the general public would do well to ask themselves this question: *How much honest optimism would you have if you knew your son or daughter was infected?*

CHAPTER 8 REFERENCES

1. Anonymous. Needlestick transmission of HTLV-III from a patient infected in Africa. Lancet 2:1376, 1984.

2. Cooper DA, Maclean P, Ginlayson R, et al. Acute AIDS retrovirus infection: Definition of a clinical illness associated with seroconversion. Lancet 1:537, 1985.

3. Fisher AG, Collati E, Ratner L, et al. A molecular clone of HTLV-III with biological activity. Nature 316:262, 1985.

4. Gallo RC. Pathogenic human retroviruses: Past, present, and Future. Unpublished remarks. August 28, 1985.

5. Groopman JE, Salahuddin SZ, Sarngadharan MG, et al. HTLV- III in saliva of people with AIDS-Related Complex and healthy homosexual men at risk for AIDS. Science 226:447, 1984.

6. Zagury D, Bernard J, Leibowitch J, et al. HTLV-III in cells cultured from semen of two patients with AIDS. Science 226:449, 1984.

7. Gallo RC, Salahuddin SZ, Popovic M, et al. Frequent detection and isolation of cytopathic retroviruses (HTLV-III) from patients with AIDS and at risk for AIDS. Science 224:500, 1984.

8. Anderson DJ, Yurris EJ. "Trojan Horse" leukocyte as in AIDS. N Engl J Med 309:985, 1983.

9. Shearer GM, Rabson AS. Semen and AIDS. Nature 308:230, 1984.

10. Stewart GJ, Cunningham AL, Driscoll GL, et al. Transmission of human T-cell lymphotropic virus type III (HTLV-III) by artificial insemination by donor. Lancet 2:581, 1985.

11. Salahuddin SZ, Groopman JE, Markham PD, et al.

HTLV-III in symptom free seronegative persons. Lancet 2:1418, 1984.

12. Harris C, Small DB, Klein RS, et al. Immunodeficiency in female sexual partners of men with the acquired immunodeficiency syndrome. N Engl J Med 308:1181, 1983.

13. Leibowitch J (Howard, R. trans.) A Strange Virus of Unknown Origin. Ballantine Books, New York, P. 57-58, 1985.

14. Alter HJ, Eichberg JW, Masur H, et al. Transmission of HTLV-III infection from human plasma to chimpanzees: An animal model for AIDS. Science 226:549, 1984.

15. McClure H, Swenson B, King F, et al. Experimental infection of chimpanzees with lymphadenopathy-associated virus. Medical Morbid Weekly Rep 33:442, 1984.

16. Scott GB, Fishl M, Klimas N, et al. Mothers of infants with the acquired immunodeficiency syndrome (AIDS): Outcomes of subsequent pregnancies (abst). International Conference on Acquired Immunodeficiency Syndrome (AIDS). Atlanta, GA, April 14-17, 1985, p. 21.

17. Saxinger WC, Levine PH, Dean AG, et al. Evidence for exposure to HTLV-III in Uganda before 1973. Science 227:1036, 1985.

18. Drotman CP. Insect-borne transmission of AIDS? JAMA 254:1085, 1985.

19. Biggar RJ, Melbye M, Sarin PS, et al. ELISA HTLV retrovirus antibody reactive associated with malaria and immune complexes in healthy Africans. Lancet 2:520, 1985.

20. Bye LL, Henne JC, Quarles RC. Designing an effective AIDS prevention campaign for San Francisco: Results from the first probability sample of an urban gay male community (abst). International Conference on Acquired Immunodeficiency Syndrome (AIDS). Atlanta, GA, April 14-17, 1985, p. 61.

21. Wong-Staal F, Shaw GM, Hahn BH, et al. Genomic di-

versity of human T-lymphotropic virus type III (HTLV-III). Science 229:759, 1985.

22. Fischinger, DJ, Bolognesi DP. Prospects for diagnostic tests, intervention, and vaccine. In *AIDS: Etiology, Diagnosis, Treatment,* and *Prevention.* DeVita VT, Hellman S, Rosenberg SA (eds). J.B. Lippincott Company, New York, p. 55-88, 1985.

23. Kovacs JA, Hiemenz JW, Macher AM, et al. *Pneumocystis carinii* pneumonia: A comparison in patients with the acquired immune deficiency syndrome and patients with other immunodeficiencies. Ann Intern Med 100:663, 1984.

24. Goedert JJ, Blattner WA. The epidemiology of AIDS and related conditions. In *AIDS: Etiology, Diagnosis, Treatment,* and *Prevention.* DeVita VT, Hellman S, Rosenberg SA (eds). J.B. Lippincott Company, New York, p. 1-30, 1985.

9

Shock Waves

Blood Tests for the AIDS Virus

One of the most valuable results of the scientific efforts to identify the AIDS virus as the cause of AIDS was the development of technology to test blood for AIDS virus antibodies. When a foreign germ invades the blood, the body's immune system prepares a new defense. Part of the defense is the production of antibodies. The antibodies are all specific for the type of germ that has invaded. For example, if a child has measles, the blood produces antibodies that specifically fight measles.

The presence of antibodies specific to the AIDS virus suggests that an individual has been infected. In certain situations, most notably in the period of latency between infection and the production of measurable antibodies, it is possible that an antibody test will not detect infection. Obviously a test that detects the virus itself would be preferable to one that detects antibodies to the virus. A number of theoretical and practical obstacles stand in the way of developing a reliable test for the virus itself. One is not likely to be available for several years.

Current testing for the AIDS virus is accomplished through a sequence of tests for antibody to the AIDS virus. The ELISA test is the most widely available tool. ELISA is an acronym for "enzyme-linked immunosorbent assay." The ELISA is almost always the initial test performed on a blood sample that is being investigated for possible AIDS virus infection. Blood samples that react negatively on the initial ELISA test are considered uninfected; in this case the test is not repeated.

The ELISA test is extremely sensitive—it will almost always react positively to blood that has been infected. However, it is so sensitive that it also reacts positively to some blood that has not actually been infected with the AIDS virus. This is due to reaction with blood-borne proteins that share similarities to the AIDS virus antibody. When a test incorrectly reacts positively to uninfected blood, it is referred to as a "false positive" outcome.

During 1984 and the early part of 1985, there was a great deal of discussion about the significance of false positive outcomes. Advocates of high-risk groups and civil liberties advocates argued strongly against the use of AIDS virus blood test results for nonmedical purposes because of the possibility of false positive outcomes. They argued that it was improper to stigmatize someone on the basis of a test that can be faulty. Fortunately, these false positive outcomes can be practically eliminated by a sequence of laboratory steps, which are now considered standard practice in AIDS virus blood testing.

Blood that initally reacts positively to the ELISA test is not considered to be definitely infected; the test is repeated up to twice more. This procedure cuts down on many of the false positive outcomes. If a blood sample reacts negatively two out of three times to the ELISA test, it is considered to be uninfected. If it reacts positively two of three times, it is referred to as "repeatedly ELISA positive." This is not a definite indication of infection. In order to make that determination, repeatedly positive ELISA blood is subjected to Western blot analysis.

The Western blot is more expensive, more difficult to run, and not as widely available as the ELISA test. It is an extremely specific test and does not have the larger number of false positive results which the ELISA has. Thus it is used to confirm repeatedly positive ELISA blood for AIDS virus infection.

Recent evidence demonstrates that the combination of ELISA and Western blot tests virtually renders concern about false positive outcomes obsolete. Any blood sample that is repeatedly ELISA positive and is confirmed by a positively Western blot test can be confidently said to be infected with the AIDS virus. Information from the first 1.6 million pints of screened donated blood indicate that repeating the ELISA test will eliminate 70% of the false positive outcomes and Western blot will eliminate the other 30%.[1]

Dr. Robert Gallo has stated that blood which is "triple positive" can be said to be infected in "999 cases out of 1,000." Recent scientific study also points unambiguously to the same conclusions. This sequence, which is now uniformly utilized for testing blood for the AIDS virus, can definitely be said to be 99+% accurate, which makes it more reliable than a number of other accepted diagnostic tests.

The development of a reliable sequence of tests by which AIDS virus infection can be detected is an important accomplishment. As a result of screening of donated blood, which began in April 1985, our nation's blood supply has been rendered a great deal safer from AIDS virus contamination. However, the fact that an accurate test exists opens up a virtual "Pandora's box" of social, ethical, and legal questions which are far from being answered.

The government has recognized this in present policies that are aimed at preserving confidentiality of test results.

Dr. Frank Young, Commissioner of Food and Drugs, wrote in a cover letter to a May 1985 mailing to American physicians: "Physicians and other health professionals should recognize the need for assuring confidentiality of test results because disclosure could lead to serious social and employment consequences. Loss of employment or insurability may occur if positive test results become a part of the medical records."

This suggestion is expanded in the body of the mail-out in a set of recommendations endorsed by the Centers for Disease Control, the National Institutes of Health, and the Drug Abuse Administration. "Screening procedures (for donated blood) should be designed with safeguards to protect disclosure.... Facilities should consider developing contingency plans in the event that disclosure is sought through the legal process." Civil liberties advocates can no longer justifiably argue that an accurate test to determine infection with the AIDS virus does not exist. The focus of arguments about the rights of infected individuals will properly shift to questions such as these: "Who should be permitted access to AIDS virus blood test results? What limitations, if any, should be placed on infected individuals?"

AIDS VIRUS INFECTION—EFFECT ON THE INDIVIDUAL

The First Dilemma—To Know or Not to Know?

The development of an accurate AIDS virus blood test opens the door for responsible individuals to determine whether or not they have been infected. Confidentiality precautions currently in place make knowledge of a positive outcome on the AIDS virus blood test sequence less damaging now than it may be at some point in the future.

Current estimates indicating 1 to 2 million Americans are infected imply that many more have been exposed without infection having taken place. There has been some confusion about the difference between "exposure" and "infection." Medically, exposure is any opportunity for the AIDS virus to enter a new bloodstream; infection is when it actually enters a new bloodstream.

This semantic discrepancy is due in part to inaccurate reporting on the AIDS epidemic. In an Associated Press report of June 1985 about notification of infected Red Cross donors, the following semantic error was made: "Scientists have estimated that as many as 1 million Americans may have been *exposed* to the virus...." The more accurate term was used by Dr. Bolognesi in his Congressional testimony: "....as many as 2 million people have already been *infected* with this deadly virus...." If there are 1 to 2 million infected with the AIDS virus, millions more have been exposed. Anyone who had sexual contact or shared a needle with an infected individual could be said to have been "exposed."

One interesting insight into the difference between exposure and infection is provided by examining the difference between government "high risk" and "at risk" categories. The Centers for Disease Control identifies the following groups as "high risk" for developing AIDS: male homosexuals or bisexuals, intravenous drug users, hemophiliacs, transfusion recipients, and sexual contacts of members of these groups.

It is notable that a much larger segment of the American population is considered to be "at risk" for developing AIDS. The Public Health Service, in the March 1985 AIDS bulletin under a heading entitled, "A Special Note To Persons Who May Be At Increased Risk for AIDS," recommends that members of the following groups refrain from donating blood due to possible AIDS virus infection: males who have had sex with one or more males since 1979, males whose sexual partner has had sex with one or more males since 1979, Haitians who entered the United States after 1977, and sexual partners of persons in these groups. The classification of "males whose sexual partner has had sex with one or more men since 1979" and "sexual partners of persons in these groups" includes nearly all sexually active heterosexuals.

It is understandable that the government err on the side of caution in protecting the nation's blood supply. This precaution demonstrates clearly that for every infected individual there are a number of other individuals who should consider themselves to be "at risk" for being infected. Certainly, any male who has sexual contact with an urban prostitute and any female who has sexual contact with a bisexual man should realize that these represent possible exposures to the AIDS virus. Accordingly, individuals who suspect that they may be infected will have to wrestle with the personal decision as to whether or not they want to get their blood tested.

The question, "Should I get my blood tested?" is the beginning of an emotionally laden series of personal crises that might be characterized under the general heading "AIDS anxiety." The hysteria that was observed in the late 1970s relating to the spread of herpes will be a fraction of what will occur as the result of the spread of the AIDS virus.

There are compelling reasons that individuals should want to know their blood status just as there are reasons why they might not. Knowing one's blood status allows one to plan for the future. Infected individuals might want to buy extra insurance while it is available without a blood test. They may also consider the implications of infection on career choice. Some careers, including the military and the health care fields may place restrictions on infected individuals. Also, infected individuals should take precautions to protect their sexual partners, reevaluate marital plans, and eliminate the idea of conceiving children. Finally, infected individuals can be particularly aware of general health habits which may reduce the risk of developing AIDS.

The reasons "not to know" are also persuasive. The question of emotional stress as a possible cofactor for the development of AIDS is being investigated. It is also possible that knowing one has been infected will have eventual legal implications. Knowing that one has a potentially fatal germ which can be transmitted sexually puts an individual in a situation where control of sexuality is imperative. Anecdotal evidence from areas of high prevalence of AIDS virus infection suggests that many will not want to know their blood status. "I guess I'm just fatalistic about it," explained one admittedly promiscuous New York gay man. "The way I see it, you get it or you don't."

Getting one's blood tested for the AIDS virus is one tangible step an individual can take to demonstrate a sense of concern about the AIDS epidemic. At present it is a voluntary step, and in 49 states there are no "strings" attached. (Colorado voted to make AIDS virus infection reportable to the health department.) Unfortunately, making the mature decision to have one's blood tested is not the only obstacle to overcome. For a responsible individual who suspects that they may be infected and would like to know, there are a number of other difficulties. Current government policies limit the use of the AIDS virus blood test.

There are three basic ways currently available by which individuals can have their blood tested for the AIDS virus. They are: by donating blood, by utilizing an "alternate test site," and by request of a physician. A symptomless individual who is not a male homosexual, intravenous drug user, prostitute, or recent immigrant from the Caribbean or central Africa is presented with a mine field of obstacles which must be overcome before the blood test can be run.

When one donates blood, the donation is now checked for AIDS virus infection by the Red Cross and individuals are personally notified if they are "triple positive" (repeatedly positive on ELISA and confirmed by a positive Western blot). Individuals tempted to ally their fears by having their blood tested courtesy of the Red Cross should know that anyone who suspects he or she may be infected is specifically requested not to donate. This list has already been described and inferentially includes most single people. This is because there is a small percentage of "false negative" results, i.e., cases of infected blood that escape detection. The use of such blood could result in both legal complications for the company whose test it escaped and medical complications for the recipient. Thus individuals who wish the blood test be run because they fear infection are directed to an "alternate site" for testing.

State health agencies have established, as of July 31, 1985, 573 alternate test sites for the AIDS virus blood test in 41 states.[1] These are to provide an option for worried individuals who might otherwise donate blood to find out if they have been infected with the AIDS virus. Alternate-site testing is a worthwhile concept, and in the future it may provide a great resource in identifying the symptomless, infected individuals.

In their first few months of operation, though, alternate test sites were more effective at convincing people not to have their blood tested than they were at encouraging participation in this important public health initiative. Individuals who called a site wishing to have his or her blood tested were first asked about inclusion in a "high risk" category. Those who admitted that they were not a male homosexual or bisexual, intravenous drug user, hemophiliac, prostitute, or recent Caribbean or central African immigrant report being discouraged from having the test done. The "inaccuracy" of the test was cited by test-site personnel, particularly the possibility of a "false positive" outcome. This argument, as we know, is misleading. Without a repeatedly positive ELISA test confirmed by a positive Western blot, no blood was to be identified as having been infected.

While doubts over false positives may have discouraged some of the alternate-site test inquiries from having the test done, another factor was the fear that positive test results would not be kept confidential. In truth, confidentiality is insured by the use of coded numbers (as opposed to names) in identifying samples. However, many inquiring high-risk individuals (mostly urban gay males) were apparently fearful of the bureaucratic procedure of having to submit to one or more "counseling sessions" which alternate sites generally require before blood is tested. For every eight inquiries in the first two months of operation, an average of two pretest counseling sessions were held. For every two counseling sessions, one blood test was performed.

Unless major changes are implemented, the vast majority of infected, symptomless individuals will continue to remain unaware of their infection. The Red Cross only expects to notify 1,600 donors in a 12-month period that they have been infected with the AIDS virus.[1] Alternate sites as they currently are set up will identify a few thousand more. In the first 10 weeks of alternate site testing in Massachusetts, for example, only 12 infected individuals were identified. With more than 1 million infected symptomless individuals, the identification of even 10,000 would be the slightest tip of a huge iceberg.

Despite this shortcoming, the state public health agencies which led the way in making alternate sites available should be commended for this public health initiative. The fact that symptomless, persistent individuals can have their blood tested and the results kept confidential is an important first step in slowing the spread of AIDS virus infection. However, until facilities such as these are not only available but widely utilized, the unchecked growth rate in AIDS virus infection will continue. The effectiveness of this initiative will depend on the willingness of "at risk" individuals to take this frightening but worthwhile step.

One of the reasons this resistance to taking the blood test will likely remain high is the desire to avoid the emotional stress previously characterized as "AIDS anxiety." This has been qualitatively described by ARC patient Johnny Greene, writing about his preoccupation with the signs and symptoms of AIDS. He tells of a life of paranoia, waking up to check if he has night sweats, looking for the appearance of purple spots on his body, and trying to fight off AIDS with his willpower.

The emotional stress of today's ARC patients may give us some clue as to the problems experienced by the identified symptomless carriers of tomorrow. Knowing that one has been infected by the AIDS virus will no doubt cause a major shift in personal perceptions for the individual. In one study[2] of homosexual or bisexual men there was a noticeable increase in physician visits (from 1 to 20 additional visits per year) related to the fear of developing AIDS. No significant differences were found between the experimental and control subjects on the basis of age, race, salary, or promiscuity. Important differences were found in statistically significant measures of depression, anxiety, preoccupation with physical appearance, and phobic concerns.

One study[3] of adult male hemophiliacs also showed a tremendous emotional stress resulting from perceived susceptibility to AIDS virus attack. One group was identified as having ARC and the other was a control group. The ARC group showed statistically significant increase (over a six-month period) in the following measurements—chronic tension, premorbid pessimism, future despair, social alienation, somatic anxiety, life threat reaction, and emotional vulnerability. The study mentioned that "particular attention should be addressed to the possible similarity of reactions between patients with a positive HTLV-III (AIDS virus) blood test and those in the experimental group."

Individuals who find out that they have been infected by the AIDS virus will no doubt undergo chronic emotional stress, probably similar to that just described. The need for counseling these individuals was mentioned by Dr. Gerald Sandler, associate vice president of the American Red Cross, as being the most costly anticipated aspect of implementing nationwide blood screening. When one considers that less than 1 out of 1,000 of those screened will prove to be infected, this statement gives an idea of the costs of providing adequate counseling.

AIDS-Virus-Positive People and Family Planning

The knowledge that one is infected with the AIDS virus will have profound and in some cases shattering effect on an individual's future plans. This cannot be demonstrated any more dramatically than in the area of family planning. The married or single person who becomes aware of his or her infection with the virus will be faced with a series of unpleasant but necessary choices.

For married individuals, knowledge of AIDS virus infection will mandate a serious change in the sexual part of marriage. If either husband or wife is found to be infected, the couple should either abstain from sexual relations or else practice some form of "safe sex." Indefinite postponement of further pregnancy will change the nature of the married couple's relationship in many cases.

How to tell one's partner about AIDS virus infection is another unpleasant topic. Information from the male homosexual community on the traumatic impact of telling one's conjugal partner of infection with the AIDS virus demonstrates that this scene is fraught with fear, anger, and blame. There is a natural curiosity and suspicion as to the reason for infection. Married people who learn of their infection will often be able to make an educated guess as to their source of infection. What they tell their mates (and what their mates will be inclined to believe) may be another story entirely.

The herpes spread creates stories of herpetic infection being a cause for the initiation of divorce proceedings. Clearly it was not picked up from the proverbial toilet seat. Because the AIDS virus cannot be transmitted from casual contact, it will be difficult to make a case for total innocence. Infection with the AIDS virus may become the grounds for divorce for any number of reasons. Infection may be presented as *de facto* proof of infidelity (or drug abuse). A second possibility is that since infection would summarily end safe conjugal relations, a divorce may be granted on that basis. Finally, a divorce may be granted on the danger the uninfected spouse realizes in terms of health.

How will marriages stand up under the strain of identified infection? A number of cases have already been observed in the marriages of hemophiliacs who learned of unexpected infection. Married couples have had to cope with the fear that both may become infected through sexual contact as well as the knowledge that natural children should not be conceived. Reports of AIDS cases among hemophiliacs have resulted in fear among friends, family, and coworkers of contracting the disease. This can lead to social isolation for the married couple and their children, cutting them off from the normal support network that develops in response to serious illness. Knowledge of infection or actual symptoms in married hemophiliacs also brings about a sense of helplessness, anger, and even rage. Infection via contaminated blood or blood products carries with it the implication of "blamelessness" for infection.

Couples whose marriage is interrupted by sexually transmitted AIDS virus infection will have a different connotation. The uninfected spouse will have to simultaneously cope with fear for the health of the spouse, fear that he or she may already be infected, and hurt at evidence of infidelity. It would not be surprising to find that married individuals will display an extreme reluctance to voluntarily have their blood tested. One would expect that the desire to avoid just such an unpleasant scene will mean that most married people who are infected will only find out if they are checked by a doctor for signs or symptoms of ARC or AIDS.

Married bisexual men, married men who utilize the services of urban prostitutes, and adulterous married women (particularly in the vicinity of large urban areas) are all at risk for contracting the AIDS virus. The most likely current scenario involves a married man who is secretly bisexual and becomes infected through homosexual contact. It is also possible that an adulterous wife could become infected via sexual contact with a bisexual man. A third possibility is that of a married man who becomes infected as a result of heterosexual contact with a prostitute. There is a growing reservoir of infection among urban prostitutes, and men who utilize their services run the risk of infection.

No matter what the source of infection, or the strategy followed by the infected spouse, one thing is clear. If one or both of a married couple is infected with the AIDS virus, a pregnancy should absolutely be ruled out. A pregnant woman is at increased risk for developing AIDS (if she is infected with the AIDS virus). Further, she can transmit the virus to an unborn child directly (through the placenta) or to an infant indirectly (through infected mother's milk). The rapidly growing number of pediatric AIDS cases is one of the most tragic aspects of the AIDS crisis. For infected parents to consider a pregnancy is to put the mother and unborn infant in a life-threatening situation. Couples currently considering having children would be wise to have an AIDS virus blood test before conceiving.

AIDS virus infection will undoubtedly change the plans of affected couples. Some may opt for adoption and some may opt for divorce (particularly if one of the spouses is uninfected). The question of adoption will be complicated by the possibility of subjecting an adopted child to the trauma of a foster parent developing AIDS at some point in the future. It is also conceivable that AIDS-virus-positive people will eventually be prevented from adopting for reasons of medical uncertainty. In the case of children already in the family, the question arises of what to tell them. Even if parents decide not to worry their children, the infection of one or both parents will place a tremendous strain on the process of raising a family.

At some point it is conceivable that some sort of license will be required by the state or federal government in order to qualify to have children. The thought of such a requirement is no doubt shocking. But if this relatively small portion of the AIDS epidemic (less than 2% of the AIDS cases have been pediatric AIDS) becomes a growing problem, voices will clamor for this step. We accept that we must be licensed to marry, to run a business, or to drive a car. Will the day arrive when we must apply for the right to have children? Will a cottage industry develop to deliver babies to infected mothers who are willing to run the risk? Will the AIDS virus cause a large increase in the already booming black market in healthy babies? None of these possibilities is out of the question.

As distressing as the personal crises that are thrust upon married infected individuals, the choices of single infected individuals (sure to be a much larger group) are no more attractive. The initial dilemma ("to know or not to know") is similar. Upon learning of infection, single people find that the world in which they live has been drastically altered.

One of the first natural questions is, "How did I get infected?" Evidence from homosexual AIDS patients suggests that this search will be filled with remorse, guilt, and self-flagellatory anger. Individuals who decide to have their blood tested will likely be doing it for the reason that they have reason to suspect infection. In some cases this may boil down to a small number of possible moments of exposure. If the point at which infection took place can even be guessed at, the question of notifying all sexual partners since that point in time comes up. Who should be told? What should they be told? Since this would be a rather excruciating exercise for an individual, perhaps in the future this sort of function will be performed by the community support systems that are developing in response to the AIDS crisis.

Promiscuity has been correlated to infection via sexual transmission. Promiscuous AIDS patients have evidenced guilt upon learning of their condition and reflect on the behavior that apparently led to it. Five reactions[4] to this guilt have been observed: 1) abstinence; 2) denial or rejection of facts leading to continued high levels of sexual activity; 3) abstinence with close friends while engaging in multiple anonymous sexual contacts; 4) increased use of drugs and alcohol; and 5) development of small groups of sexual contacts. It would not be surprising to see a similar pattern of reaction by AIDS-virus-positive people to knowledge of infection.

In any case, a single infected individual will operate in a seriously restricted world. Conceiving natural children should be ruled out. The only form of marriage that should be considered is one in which some form of "safe sex" is practiced, ad infinitum. It is hard to imagine many couples settling for that kind of future.

As with the herpes spread, the appearance of quiet, confidential AIDS-virus-positive dating services would not be a surprising development. The possibility of coinfection with a different variant of the virus or another sexually transmitted disease would make arrangements like this less than desirable. How will the infected single person cope with the kind of stress that knowledge of infection will create? Probably by acting as many urban gay men have. There seems to be a pattern of "settling down" with a monogamous partner, minimizing risks by use of condoms and "safe sex," and trying to live as normal a life as possible. A life of waiting for the medical miracle that may never come to pass and thinking back on the momentary bliss of fulfilled lust will undoubtedly be a part of the sadness of the infected single person.

The day when there are millions of young, single infected people in America may soon be upon us. Once identified, these people may frequently have contemplative, depressed existences. Stigmatized by the impracticality of marriage or conceiving children, facing an uncertain medical future, AIDS-virus-positive people will find that infection has put many of the powers of choice out of their hands.

For the uninfected single person the chance of joining the ranks of the infected on a "one-night stand" hardly seems to be worth the risk. The AIDS virus may well take a lot of the joy out of lustful, anonymous sex and replace it with a manic, desperate, self-destructive quality. Groucho Marx once said that he wouldn't want to join any country club that would have him as a member. The promiscuous single person would do well to apply that kind of thinking to the choice of sexual partners. With each partner representing a "roll of the dice," the guilt and anxiety that accompanies casual sex may well lead to fewer and fewer sexual adventures. (Perhaps more appropriate than rolling a die is taking another chance on a game of Russian roulette.) With symptomless carriers making up the vast majority of infected individuals, the possibility that this next partner may represent a source of infection may cause drastic revision in personal sexual habits. In observing the drastic change of homosexual men, psychologist Steven Morin said, "There seems to be an association between sexual activities and death, and that is creating less sexual interest."

Will the next decade or two witness a serious rollback of the era of permissiveness which we have been experiencing since the middle of the 1960s? Will there be a "new morality" based more on pragmatic self-interest than scriptural teaching? Will single people be able to adjust to the new realities created by the AIDS virus? It is not too dramatic to say that their lives, their careers, their happiness, and their potential legacies absolutely depend on it.

AIDS-Virus-Positive People—Personal Planning

AIDS-virus-infection may be an influence that significantly alters career paths. As with many other AIDS-related issues, the effect that infection will have on career plans will be directly related to the long-term natural history of infection. Important statistical indices will be the morbidity (serious medical complications) and mortality (death rate) at 5, 10, 15, 20 and 25 years. If the medical prognosis for AIDS-virus-positive people shows increasingly dramatic morbidity and mortality, for example, at 10 years it is conceivable there will be dramatic career shifts by infected individuals. Facing the prospect of a shortened life span, infected people may tend to forgo higher education and more seriously consider a career option in which it is possible to make one's mark rather early.

Certainly one aspect of the AIDS-virus-positive individual's life should be assiduous attention to sound basic health and diet habits. The evidence on the importance of "cofactors" in triggering an active phase of AIDS virus infection is now under way. It does seem as though infected people who have poor health habits and chronic illness are at greater risk for developing AIDS than otherwise healthy individuals. The infected individual should take extra care to observe "common sense" rules of good health—plenty of rest, a balanced diet, moderate, regular exercise, and the avoidance of nonprescribed drugs, smoking, and alcohol. Since there is speculation that antigenic stimulation can encourage AIDS virus replication, infected individuals should take particular care to guard against further infection of all kinds.

On a personal level the life of an AIDS-virus-positive person will be filled with a gnawing sense of doubt. Although the distinction between full-blown AIDS and AIDS-related complex has been consistently made in this text, the distinction is not so clear to many of the victims of AIDS-related complex. These people have experienced an obvious attack on their immune system, and to many the inevitability of AIDS seems quite real. In fact, the rather inexact term "pre-AIDS" is often used by these people to indicate this sense of preordination. When symptomless carriers are identified in great numbers, it would not be surprising to witness a modified version of this type of reaction.

The question of how to cope with this life of stress and uncertainty is likely to produce a large array of answers. There may be a reemergence of the kind of "consciousness raising" groups that became popular in the 1970's. Techniques such as Transcendental Meditation, Scientology, astrology, Zen Buddhism, Rolfing, and a variety of other attempts at inducing tranquility may become common in infected individuals.

Gay communities have set up model programs such as hospices and support groups to help people cope with AIDS. These no doubt will take place on a large scale as the disease becomes more prevalent and may eventually expand to include all infected individuals. It is also likely that some will turn to alcohol and drugs for stimulation and distance from reality.

Prudent estate planning may be an unpleasant but necessary part of an infected person's overall game plan. Individuals with shortened life spans should consider the postmortem consequences of their financial decisions. These include the advantages and disadvantages of joint ownership, appropriate beneficiary designation in life insurance, pension, and profit-sharing plans, reevaluation of present assets, and the necessity for a legal, up-to-date will.

There are many stories about young AIDS patients planning their own funeral services, burial, or cremation. The reluctance of morticians to embalm dead AIDS patients continues to be a problem. Euthanasia and suicide may come to be viewed by some as a justifiable response in end-stage AIDS patients, no doubt raising the deep philosophical questions that accompany them.

Depending on how they choose to react, AIDS-virus-positive people may become a great resource for society, contributing with intensity and commitment with the prospect of a shortened life span. On the other hand, many may exhibit residual bitterness, vengefulness, lethargy, and alienation. How much of this will come to pass? As of this writing, more than 6,000 Americans have died of AIDS. In the next five years it is expected that 15 times that many will die. The shock waves caused already by the AIDS virus in many urban homosexual communities are a hint of what a much larger segment of America will soon begin to witness.

EFFECT ON SOCIETY

Preventing the Spread of Infection

The Role of Education

With the prospect of an effective vaccine for the AIDS virus apparently five years or more in the future, efforts to slow the spread of AIDS virus infection will be a combination of educational measures and epidemiological restrictions. Many of the epidemiological measures that would be effective would involve a degree of governmental interference many would regard as excessive. Voluntary measures are clearly preferable.

The budget of the federal government reflects an increased awareness of the need for public dissemination of information. In fiscal year 1984, at a total of $964,000 (2%) of a $51 million AIDS budget was dedicated to public dissemination of information. In fiscal year 1985, $3.8 million (4%) of a $93 million budget was dedicated to this. In the revised budget proposal for 1986, $21.7 million (11%) of a $196 million budget was allocated for this purpose.

The Department of Health and Human Services, after much prodding, has recognized education as the only viable means of slowing the spread of AIDS virus infection. However, this appropriation of $21.7 million should also be compared with the growing size of the AIDS problem. If Dr. Bolognesi is correct, 2 million Americans will become infected for the first time in the 12-month period between July 1985 and July 1986. Even if that number were quartered, the infection of 500,000 Americans will likely create 25,000–100,000 new AIDS cases and 125,000 ARC patients. The cost of caring for the AIDS patients alone will be between *$2.5 and $10 billion*. This does not include care for ARC patients or any AIDS research. Given the fact that the government will ultimately "foot the bill" for AIDS patients whose personal resources and insurance are unable to cover the high medical costs, it is clear that every effort should be made to encourage voluntary reduction of risky sexual behavior.

One of the arguments over the public dissemination of information will be the kind of information that is distributed. People will want to influence the "moral tone" of the message, depending on their political point of view. Evangelists will want the information to be explained in a manner that condemns premarital and extramarital sex. A more liberal point of view would put emphasis on the practical, preventive steps that can be taken to prevent infection.

This clash in viewpoints may boil down to the classical argument about means and ends. Do the ends (objectives) of a project justify the means (methods by which it was achieved)? This argument is not a hypothetical one. A community project that helped slow the spread of sexually transmitted disease in Houston will illustrate the dilemma.

A group of Houston health educators[5] developed a three-year, three-phase program to try and slow the spread of the virus. In the first year the focus was on the dissemination of basic information about AIDS. The objective was to make as much of the targeted community (male gays in Houston) aware that AIDS was sexually transmitted, that it affected gay men in great numbers, and that promiscuity seemed to be correlated with its development. It was hoped that this information would stimulate fear and people would change their attitude about anonymous sex and thus promiscuity would be reduced. Little change took place.

In the second year it was decided that a more drastic approach was needed. Fear did not seem to be able to produce a reduced level of promiscuity, so the group aimed at the "next best alternative." It was decided that although the information on the efficacy of "safe sex" (sex that involves no exchange of body fluids) was inconclusive, it represented a more realistic approach to promote. So the group aggressively promoted "safe sex," attempting to make *"safe sex seem acceptable, gay-positive, and palatable....*(Emphasis supplied.) This phase produced an extremely high awareness level (79%), a significant shift in attitudes (63%), and a lower but significant shift in behavior (42%).

In the third year the group decided to expand on this theme and actively merchandise the concept of "safe sex." Many modern marketing techniques were utilized to encourage the practice of "safe sex." *"Events included a Play-Safe PlayMate Contest, Playsafe themes, graphics, work-*

shops, Playsafe decorations in bars, Playsafe hankies, t-shirts, and a PlaySafe PlayMate Calendar for 1985." (Emphasis supplied.) The results of this promotion will not be known until early 1986. However, there is a significant decline in the Houston male homosexual population of *all* kinds of sexually transmitted diseases.

In this population the dissemination of the basic information was apparently not enough to cause a change in attitude or behavior. It was not until a positive alternative was promoted that change took place. A promotion on "what to do" was far more effective than a promotion on "what not to do."

Another plausible explanation is that changes in attitude and behavior had very little to do with the program. These may be more closely linked to the continued local and national growth in diagnosed AIDS cases. As more men contract AIDS and die, the community concern is bound to grow. This is only one study in one particular population. Nevertheless, it presents some of the questions that will undoubtedly come up about the kind and tone of information that should be presented.

To what extent should government get involved in the dissemination of information involving sexual practices? Should government implicitly condone and encourage sexual practices of any kind? If public funding is involved, what say should taxpayers have in the information that is distributed? If it can be proven to slow the spread of the virus and thus save lives, isn't it a good idea? Or, is this an area that government should leave alone? If public funding will ultimately pay the medical bills for the many who are victimized by AIDS, isn't this kind of information dissemination justified? Does dissemination of information on "safe sexual practices" actively promote promiscuity?

The argument will follow the same lines as the argument over the distribution of information on contraception by such organizations as Planned Parenthood. One side argues that sex among young people is a reality and therefore it makes sense to teach people how to avoid pregnancy and venereal disease. The other side contends that to distribute information about contraception is to condone and promote sexual promiscuity. To prevent an AIDS virus infection is to prevent a possible terminal illness. The stakes are quite high. What kind of information should be presented? Is "moral tone" more important than effectiveness?

The means-ends debate about information will extend to the methods of informing people beyond high-risk communities about the danger of AIDS. One of the techniques used to encourage safe driving habits is the showing of films involving the results of unsafe driving habits. Will a video "trip" to the AIDS ward be part of the AIDS preventive education package? Reformed drug addicts, convicts, and alcoholics sometimes tour high schools to warn of the dangers of young adulthood. Will AIDS patients perform similar roles? The spread of information about AIDS is bound to cause controversy. But it will not cause nearly the kind of controversy more aggressive government action will create.

Widespread Utilization of Available Alternate Test Sites

In preventing the further spread of AIDS virus infection it is hard to imagine a more important priority than the identification of those already infected. If the 1 million or more symptomless carriers could be informed of their situation, a great slowdown in the spread of infection could result from responsible sexual behavior on the part of these individuals. Although the technology exists to accurately identify infected people, it is currently sadly underutilized.

The alternate test sites have already been described. Although the "early returns" may not be indicative, it appears that this method at present will identify less than 10,000 infected individuals, or less than 1% of the total number.

How can this be changed? When a blood test is run, there is a great deal of benefit. Infected individuals can be referred for regular medical evaluation and can take measures to protect their own health as well as preventing infection of others. Uninfected individuals can gain peace of mind as well as an increased awareness of the importance of preventive measures.

There are a number of obstacles that need to be overcome in order to fully utilize alternate site testing. At the NIH meeting on July 31, 1985, one problem mentioned was funding. Many states are resistant to either reallocate existing resources or unwilling to seek additional funding for these alternate sites. Many alternate sites have a small staff and limited laboratory facilities. In many cases Western blot analysis cannot be performed. This means that repeatedly positive ELISA samples must be sent out, which greatly adds to the time between when the test is run and the results are available.

Former Secretary of Health and Human Services Margaret Heckler included in her revised budget request more than $21 million in community risk reduction–health education and demonstration and evaluation projects. Some of this money is targeted at high-risk areas and some is allocated to each state, apparently to act as "seed money" for necessary projects. One worthwhile priority is to make sure that alternate test sites are functioning effectively, at a much higher level of activity than anything seen to date.

Another obstacle is the demonstrated reluctance of individuals in high-risk groups to use these facilities. Hopefully as members of these groups learn that true confidentiality exists and there are no "hidden agendas" involved, more will have their blood tested. Certainly the leadership of these communities should encourage members to have their blood tested. The National Gay Task Force lobbied hard to have the alternate sites made available. A similar emphasis should now be placed on their use. With infection among male homosexuals estimated at 800,000 to 1.2

million, it is obvious that the results of the first few months show tremendous underutilization of these facilities.

Another major obstacle to the use of alternate test sites is bureaucratic rigmarole. People should not be forced to sit through one or more "counseling sessions" in order to have their test run. The government has implicitly testified as to the veracity of the test by claiming that the nation's blood supply has been made safe through its implementation and in approving its use by the military to screen new recruits. Since the test is reliable, its use should be encouraged. In performing these voluntary tests, the principle of confidentiality should be adhered to rigorously. Making AIDS virus infection reportable, as was done in Colorado, without strong pressures to protect the confidentiality of results from employers, insurers, and landlords, will not serve public health goals. Individuals will obviously resist having their blood tested. Individuals should be able to have the test run without name or address given—a numerical code should be a sufficient way to identify blood samples.

The American Red Cross and the other blood-collecting facilities around the country have done an excellent job in quickly implementing national screening of the 9 million units of donated blood which will be processed in the first year of the program. A potentially chaotic situation was handled with professionalism and good judgment. Federal, state, and local governments should learn from this example and make a concerted effort to encourage the widespread use of alternate site testing for the AIDS virus.

Epidemiological Restrictions

It is government's historic responsibility to preserve the public health. The use of government intervention to prevent the spread of infectious disease is a well-established principle. In 48 states a blood test is required for a marriage license. Each applicant's blood is checked for syphilis infection. If either partner or both show infection, they must be able to prove that they have been treated in order to qualify for the license. The justification for this is protection of the public health and prevention of the spread of syphilis.

More drastic measures have been taken in health emergencies. There is precedent for compulsory immunization of populations that prove to be at high risk for the development of disease (such as school children or soldiers going to tropical environments). Even more dramatic is quarantine, which has been used to prevent the spread of polio and tuberculosis.

AIDS is the first potentially fatal venereal disease to appear since World War II and the development of antibiotics. The continued epidemic spread of AIDS virus infection appears to be a virtual certainty. Among the possible tools to prevent the spread of infection are a variety of government interventions.

We have already witnessed an example of successful government action to prevent the spread of AIDS virus infection. During 1982 the first cases of transfusion-related AIDS appeared. It became apparent that the agent that caused AIDS could be transmitted through the transfusion of infected blood. The government acted in 1983 to protect the nation's blood supply by urging members of identified high-risk groups to refrain from donating. In early 1985 a more dramatic step was taken. Starting May 1985, all donated blood is now screened for AIDS virus infection. This represents a large financial commitment, nearly $100 million annually, but health care professionals are in agreement that this step, however costly, was necessary to protect the nation's blood supply. One estimate predicts that this screening procedure will cost $2 million per AIDS case prevented.

There are a number of other possible government interventions that could attempt to slow the spread of AIDS virus infection. In June 1985 the *Journal of the American Medical Association* came out in an editorial for the consideration of the AIDS virus blood test as a marital screen.

This would be a drastic step, as it would mean preventing (not merely delaying) marriages. It would likely be of little value in preventing the spread of infection. By the time a couple has applied for a marriage license, the likelihood that the relationship has not been "consummated" is rather small. Those few couples who have sexually abstained prior to their marriage are highly unlikely to be infected.

A more dramatic suggestion would be the requirement of the AIDS virus blood test in order to conceive children. A law that attempted to license childbearing would be quite difficult to enforce. What would represent appropriate penalties and enforcement procedures? Laws that are difficult to enforce do exist (such as laws against marijuana use and prostitution) and as such are more useful as "goals." One expert on legal control of sexually transmitted disease has described the difficulties in enforcing reporting laws. In cases such as these, the law is useful as a goal, and enforcement can be applied in cases of blatant, willful disregard.

Another epidemiological approach would be to aggressively crack down on likely sources of contagion—such as gay bathhouses and houses of prostitution. Closing of the gay bathhouses has almost been accomplished already without government interference. Many have closed due to decreased business in response to fear of AIDS. In Washington, D.C., the number of gay bathhouses has dropped from six to one in the last three years. Owners point out that safe sex guidelines are prominent, condoms are available, and that places such as this are preferable alternatives to other places for clandestine sex. Nevertheless, the practice of "unsafe sex" takes place at gay bathhouses. Pediatric AIDS specialist Dr. James Oleske said, "Bathhouses are dens of iniquity—they're places where infection spreads."

Prostitutes have been shown to facilitate the spread of the AIDS virus in Africa and likely are infected in large numbers in America. However, since prostitution is illegal in 49 states it is difficult to gain access to a large segment of the prostitute population. Many cities have had periods of "crackdown" on prostitution, which are then followed by a return to a state of normalcy. An approach that licensed prostitutes (subject to regular blood testing) might help in slowing the spread of AIDS virus infection. However, the practical question of what to do with infected prostitutes who continue to practice their trade remains. Also, this would require a massive revision of state and city laws, and thus this approach may prove to be neither practical nor effective.

Another approach would be to make AIDS virus infection a disease that must be reported to the public health department. Any health care professional who diagnoses a reportable disease is required to send a form to the local health department. The information required depends on applicable law, which varies state by state and disease by disease. In certain cases all that is necessary is to report the fact that the disease has been diagnosed. Certain states insist (for some diseases) on including identifying information such as the patient's name, address, and Social Security number.

Currently AIDS is reportable in 45 states and the District of Columbia. The CDC requests that individuals with AIDS be identified by name, and information is kept at the local health department. A computerized code is used between the health department and the CDC. The issue of confidentiality in reporting is extremely sensitive. There is a generally accepted health precept allowing an individual to control access to his or her medical records. There is a competing right of government to protect the general welfare of its citizens. The idea of making AIDS virus infection reportable highlights this conflict.

Gay-rights and civil-liberties advocates argue against this step. Fears have been expressed that the names of infected individuals could be released with dire consequences for them. Listed among the concerns are restrictions in housing, employment, insurance, and prosecution on the basis of sodomy statutes (still on the books in 23 states).

There are also persuasive public health arguments in favor of making AIDS virus infection a reportable disease. Infected individuals should be fully informed about measures they can take to reduce the risk of transmitting the virus to others. They should also have regular medical follow-up evaluation. Additionally, the study of the health patterns in symptomless, infected individuals may help in the efforts to better understand the actual pattern of AIDS virus infection.

The Colorado Board of Health voted to make AIDS virus infection (as determined by a positive AIDS virus blood test) reportable. The nine-member Colorado board of health voted unanimously to approve this step, which will become law on October 30. This sort of step may be taken by other states. Kristin Gebbie, former president of the Oregon State Health Officials, said, "More of the states are talking about it. Colorado just got their plan organized ahead of the rest of us."

While initiatives such as this are intended to protect the public health, they will have the unfortunate consequence of discouraging people from having their blood tested. The stated purpose of the Colorado initiative is to insure that infected individuals get proper follow-up and counseling about preventive measures to reduce the risk of transmitting the virus to others. However, it was not made clear why such counseling and follow-up should be done on an involuntary basis.

There are two possible ways to overcome this problem. One way would be to attach some incentive to having one's blood tested. This might include free or reduced-rate medical care, access to experimental therapies if the disease develops, or some combination of the two. A more severe approach would be to mandate screening, either at targeted groups or the general population.

Precedent exists for involuntary immunization of identifiable high-risk groups, such as schoolchildren or soldiers going to an area of high disease. However, immunization is far different from involuntary screening. It is an act that protects the individual against disease. Involuntary screening for the AIDS virus blood test would provide no immediate, tangible medical benefits to the infected individual. Since both homosexuality and use of nonprescription intravenous drugs are illegal in many states, it would be nearly impossible to gain systematic access to members of these "high risk" populations.

The other option would be to mandate AIDS virus blood test screening for all adults. This would of course be quite an expensive proposition. In order to effectively utilize national screening to stop AIDS virus infection, it would have to be performed on a regular basis for a period of time (perhaps every six months for two to three years). Additionally, to be effective there would have to be some method of curtailing the sexual activity of infected members.

There are two methods of control that are currently used with sexually transmitted diseases. *Contact tracing* involves getting in touch with recent sexual partners of infected individuals. The authority to perform this sensitive procedure is assumed by the state in order to break up a "chain of infection." Contact tracing is usually performed in circumstances in which infected individuals can be treated. With no effective treatment to neutralize AIDS virus infection, it is difficult to imagine what purpose contact tracing would serve, other than to aid in detailed transmission studies.

Another method of controlling infectious sexually transmitted disease is the *health hold order*, which is issued on behalf of a public health official and is covered by state law to an individual to comply with examination and treatment. Health hold orders are often issued in cases of sexual crimes, in which an individual can be held for a period of time. Once again these would be of limited applicability in controlling AIDS virus infection because there is no treatment that will render an individual uninfectious.

Short of massive quarantine (clearly impractical with more than 1 million infected people), one possible approach might involve mandatory national blood screening and the issuance of health identity cards, placing legal restrictions on the sexual activities of infected individuals.

It is hard to imagine this approach being attempted in a free society.

Donald Bross, J.D., Ph.D[6] analyzed the legal difficulties inherent in controlling sexually transmitted disease and developed a hypothetical three-phase plan for their control.

PHASE I

1. Enact enabling legislation to state the basic purposes, authority, and limitations of public health efforts to control sexually transmitted disease (STDs).
2. Authorize epidemiological studies by gathering confidential data to determine incidence and prevalence of STDs in each sector of the population.

PHASE II

3. Based on prior experiences, and data gathered in Phase I, establish public clinics, STD specialists, physician extender programs, or other preferred programs of intervention. Enact appropriate licensing legislation.
4. Require reporting of STDs by all professionals and paraprofessionals diagnosing or treating STDs.
5. Authorize contact tracing and health hold orders based on reasonable epidemiological suspicion of STD exposure. Expressly authorize health holds for specific groups, such as detained prostitutes, where appropriate.

PHASE III

6. Authorize physical examinations on an involuntary basis for confined cases, if this was not done previously.
7. Permit screening of epidemiologically documented high-risk groups. Note that this permits screening even when there is no specific exposure on which to form a basis for evaluation. Designate high-risk groups as appropriate.
8. Consider authorizing large-scale screening to issuance of identity cards as part of a major crackdown, if resources are available and prevalence figures warrant an effort of this degree.

It should be mentioned that this plan was conceived

before the AIDS virus had been identified. When the plan was written, there were no fatal sexually transmitted diseases. It is interesting to observe the progression some states are making in light of the various steps in the program. Steps 2, 3, and 4 are now under way in the state of Colorado and perhaps soon in other states. Step 2, the gathering of data on infection in various population segments, is part of the Centers for Disease Control response to AIDS. The development of alternate test sites is a type of physician extender program (step 3)—counselors could be described as paraprofessionals. Required reporting of AIDS virus infection (step 4) is the step recently taken by Colorado and apparently may be taken by other states in the near future. Contact tracing might be a useful way of identifying other infected members (short of mandatory screening).

It is hard to imagine a consensus developing for anything like a "Phase III" approach in America. In addition to the enormous expense, it would necessitate an intrusion of government into the private lives of Americans far beyond anything that has yet come to pass.

A less severe approach is that being taken in England, where regulations passed this year give local authorities the option to hold someone who is suspected of willingly infecting others with the AIDS virus. This provides a method of controlling the blatantly reckless infected individuals who refuse to control themselves. But it has severe drawbacks. One is the possibility that it would be selectively enforced, and thus be a tool for the oppression of individuals in high-risk groups. Another is that with so few infected individuals identified it is hard to imagine how often it could be reasonably utilized.

Restricting the spread of the AIDS virus through the implementation of epidemiological measures is fraught with difficulty. Methods that could easily be implemented such as using the blood test for a marital screen and making infection a reportable disease would likely have little effect. Measures such as policing prostitutes and closing gay bathhouses involve both legal and logistical obstacles that could not be easily overcome. Implementation of screening targeted at high-risk groups would be difficult to accomplish because individuals in these groups would be hard to identify. Mandatory national screening and the issuance of health identity cards is one approach that may have some theoretical value but would involve a great deal of expense and an incursion into the private areas of sexuality generally regarded as not the business of the state. The more plausible suggestions would probably do little to slow the spread; the approaches likely to be effective have tremendous roadblocks. After examining these options, it becomes even more clear—a voluntary wholesale revision in sexual habits is the only practical hope.

Protecting Freedoms of AIDS-Virus-Positive People

With the likelihood of 1.5 million infected people by the end of 1985 and that figure doubling each year for the rest of the decade, the problems in protecting the freedoms of AIDS-virus-positive people will become increasingly larger. The civil rights battle for AIDS-virus-positive people to date has been primarily fought by gay-rights advocates. As individuals beyond the "high risk" groups become identified in greater numbers, this battle will intensify and broaden. How can society protect the rights of infected individuals in such a way that the public health is adequately protected?

Gay-rights advocates have listed fear of housing restrictions and physical violence among possible "AIDS backlash" actions. The fact that the virus cannot be transmitted by casual contact should dictate housing policy–no individual should be denied housing because he or she is infected with the AIDS virus. The suspicion that "AIDS hysteria" will lead to physical violence will be difficult to confirm. However, the authors would like to state the obvious—VIOLENT ACTS PERPETRATED ON INDIVIDUALS BECAUSE OF A FEAR OF AIDS ARE REPUGNANT AND SHOULD BE CONDEMNED BY ALL.

Individuals who attempt to justify their violent acts by citing a fear of AIDS are demonstrating cowardice, ignorance, and bigotry.

Another concern expressed by gay-rights advocates is that AIDS-virus-positive people will be prosecuted on the basis of sodomy statutes. In 23 states certain sexual practices, among them homosexual sex, are considered a felony. (See Figure 9-1.) Recently the Fifth Circuit Court of Appeals upheld the Texas sodomy statute, based on "the strong objection to homosexual conduct, which has prevailed in Western culture for the past 7 centuries." Prosecution on the basis of violating these statutes is not common. Some of them outlaw oral-genital sex between man and wife. However, their existence places homosexual AIDS-virus-positive people in legal jeopardy.

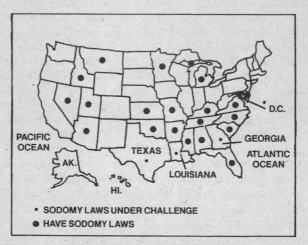

Figure 9-1. Where sodomy laws still exist.

Many of these statutes have resisted court challenges over the past several years and do not show promise of being overturned by remedial legislation. A common-sense approach might be to seek legislation that makes it illegal to prosecute for sodomy on the basis of an AIDS virus blood test. The test should not be used as *de facto* proof of homosexuality or drug abuse. Both individual good and public health good is served by identifying infected individuals. Everything possible should be done to encourage people to take the blood test.

The preservation of confidentiality of the identities of infected individuals is another area that deserves consideration. A procedure often used to protect confidentiality is "voluntary informed consent." If an AIDS virus blood test is to be run for any reason (diagnostic, blood donation screening, military screening, alternate-site testing), the individual submitting to the test should be fully informed about what will happen. He or she should be made aware of the exact procedures for handling information about test results. This should specifically include who can and cannot have access to the test result.

The Red Cross and other blood-collecting facilities around the country are scrupulously protecting the names of donors with a positive blood test for the AIDS virus. Names are kept on a deferral list, the reason for deferral is kept confidential, and only authorized individuals (those with a "need to know" for medical reasons) have access to the list. Specifically, a positive outcome is not to be released to employers, landlords, or insurance companies. These rights are protected even in Colorado, where state law calls for mandatory reporting. Alternate test sites in most states generally make use of a code number in processing blood samples, so that an individual need not feel anxious about the information being used against him or her.

A variation of the standard Red Cross procedure occurs when the donor is a member of the military. In accordance with a July 1985 agreement, the Red Cross will turn over to the military the names of any enlisted blood donors who test positively for the AIDS virus. Donors will be aware of this procedure in advance and any who opt not to donate may do so with confidentiality.

Another important issue is the confidentiality guaranteed to individuals who volunteer for a study of AIDS virus infection. This is generally covered by state law, and most states protect individuals in research projects as far as safety is concerned. The subject of protecting the information that develops about an individual during the course of the project is generally not covered. This is important because in order to determine in greater detail patterns of AIDS virus transmission, intimate questions are asked of subjects. Information about personal lives, including sexual practices and drug use, are sometimes revealed in the course of the study. The federal government should take the lead in recommending policies that can remedy this loophole in the law.

The question of how best to provide for the education of AIDS-virus-positive children is becoming an explosive issue. A great deal of national attention has been focused on Kokomo, Indiana, where hemophiliac AIDS patient Ryan White is being prevented from attending classes. The authors believe that it is incorrect to deny a youngster of this age access to the classroom because of AIDS virus infection (and, by implication, infectivity). The virus will not be transmitted to another child if simple precautions are observed. However, in a severely immune-suppressed child the exposure to the variety of germs at a public school may prove to be more detrimental to the student than the student would be to his or her classmates. This choice should be made by the student and his or her parent or guardian.

A different issue exists if the child is young, particularly of the preschool or day-care age. Children such as these do not know how to control themselves and, in vigorous play or through involuntary behavior (perhaps caused by neurological damage), may bite another child, creating a transmission opportunity. The isolation of an AIDS-virus-positive child is a regrettable step. Dr. Sheldon Landesman of the Downstate Medical Center in Brooklyn, New York, tells of one infant whose mother died of AIDS. The child had so little contact with people, according to Dr. Landesman, that it showed very little human reaction. He explained that a Cabbage Patch doll placed next to the child caused one doctor to observe that "you could hardly tell the difference between the child and the doll."

There are some difficult questions to answer with respect to the education of AIDS-virus-infected children. How should the line be drawn between those who are old enough to be responsible for their actions and those who are still too young? Should schoolchildren in areas of high prevalence be screened for AIDS virus infection? How can an infected child's right to public education be protected while protecting his or her classmates from infection?

Parents who wish to bar people with AIDS (teachers, administrators, cafeteria workers, and students) from schools should keep in mind that the large percentage of infected individuals are symptomless. Thus, in addition to those with AIDS or ARC, there are many more who are infected, presumably infectious, and symptomless. The only way to identify these people is to insist on AIDS virus blood screening. A more practical approach is to make available to infected children home tutoring, to restrict infected children below a certain age, and to encourage preventive practices.

There have been two extremely significant events relating to the freedoms of infected individuals which took place this summer. On July 31, 1985, at the National Institutes of Health meeting the government claimed that the safety of the nation's blood supply had been insured by the use of AIDS virus screening. There was strong consensus among health care professionals in attendance that the sequence already described constitutes an accurate test for AIDS virus infection. The next important event took place on August 30, 1985, when the military announced that it intended to screen applicants with the AIDS virus blood test. This represented the first use of the blood test to limit an individual's choice of career on the basis of AIDS virus infection. What will be the next profession that uses the blood test as a screening device?

It is a generally accepted principle of employment that although employees are presumed to be "engaged at will" (that is free to seek a different employment possibility at any time—and therefore that employers have latitude with respect to hiring and firing as long as blatant discrimination does not take place) they should not be denied or terminated from employment due to a physical handicap as long as it does not interfere with normal functioning on the job.

There have been examples of AIDS and ARC patients who were able to function at work but were terminated by their employer. These cases are being challenged on the grounds that their condition represents a handicap that does not interfere with job function. This is a developing area of the law. Precedents established in cases now in litigation will be important in defining the employment rights of AIDS-virus-positive individuals.

There are two responses used by employers to defend the action of firing an AIDS or ARC patient who is, temporarily at least, able to work. One is "job related" insufficiencies. ARC sufferer Johnny Greene (quoted already) was fired by McDermott, Inc., a New Orleans marine construction company shortly after his article was published in *People* magazine. A company spokesperson claimed that Greene was fired for work-related reasons.

The second grounds cited by employers is the possibility that the AIDS or ARC employee presents a health risk to the employees and customers served by the employer. A 31-year-old clerk was fired by Broward County, Florida, because he has AIDS. The ACLU is seeking $5 million in damages. Broward County has responded by saying that the clerk's doctor was unable to state unequivocally that the clerk would not infect his coworkers.

The authors believe that the evidence against casual

transmission is so strong that individuals (AIDS patients, ARC patients, AVRDS patients, and symptomless carriers) should not be restricted in employment unless the nature of their employment is such that they represent a legitimate risk to infect others. There are professions in which arguments have been made about infected individuals possibly transmitting the virus to others—health care, food preparation, and (in certain conditions) entertainment.

Is it reasonable to restrict workers in health care and food preparation on the basis of infection with the AIDS virus? Most people would not want to be in physical contact with a doctor, nurse, or dentist who is infected with the virus. A dentist, for example, might conceivably have a portal to the bloodstream when a tooth was being removed. The possibility exists for infected saliva or a small finger cut creating an avenue for transmission for the virus. Early data suggests that proper precautions in the general field of health care have cut down tremendously on the possibility of AIDS transmission. There have been few cases yet documented in this country of a needle-stick accident between an infected needle and a health care worker causing transmission of the virus. A recent National Institutes of Health study of 544 employees support the idea that proper precautions prevent accidental transmission. This, however, is from infected patient to uninfected health care worker. The possibility of an infected individual having primary patient contact on a regular basis is certainly troubling. It is equally troubling, though, to consider terminating a health care career that takes years of dedication and a large investment. Should health care workers be required to take an AIDS virus blood test? What action should be taken for infected individuals? One option would be switching to an area of health care or research that does not require primary patient contact. Current health care procedures apparently prevent AIDS virus transmission, so this might be a reasonable precaution or choice.

A similar argument could be made in the food-service industry about those in direct contact with the food being prepared. The possibility that the virus could be transmitted through this activity is quite slim. While it is conceivable that an infected individual could cut himself and a small amount of blood could end up in the prepared food, available data suggest that transmission through food preparation is unlikely to occur, especially if plastic gloves are required. The idea of screening food handlers for AIDS virus infection cannot be empirically supported.

The fear of transmission in the work place has been documented extensively in the health care field. Some health care workers have been known to want to avoid entirely all contact with AIDS patients. Even the logical presentation of the low risk of transmission due to casual contact is not persuasive enough for many. Reports abound of AIDS patients being treated like lepers in some hospitals. Since this industry is bound to be the most scientifically sophisticated, what is the likely reaction in other industries? It is not too dramatic to suggest that anyone identified as having the AIDS virus will be subject to selective treatment by his or her coworkers.

AIDS-virus-positive actors and actresses only present a risk to others if they perform in scenes that require intimate sexual contact. The news of Rock Hudson's diagnosis of AIDS has apparently created a firestorm of paranoia in the entertainment industry. Stories have circulated about actors or actresses who play in intimate scenes wishing to have their partners screened for AIDS virus infection. This is certainly a reasonable precaution. However, this does *not* mean that infected individuals should be denied opportunities for work if they do not have to play intimate scenes. There is no reason whatsoever for a general "blacklisting" of infected actors or actresses in general or male homosexual or bisexual actors in particular.

Occupations in which there could be said to be a legitimate fear of AIDS virus transmission are quite rare. The AIDS virus blood test should be utilized cautiously in those few instances in which a real transmission opportunity could be said to exist. However, even this limited use opens up a series of difficult questions. What is a reasonable way to compensate for lost wages due to a job change necessitated by infection? What are rational policies to see that the blood test is used to protect people from infection, but not abused to selectively deny employment unnecessarily?

Closely related to employment is the subject of insurance. This is considered by many volunteers who work in AIDS support groups to be the "key issue." AIDS and ARC patients who lose their jobs usually lose the health insurance plan that goes along with the job. Such measures may seriously undermine these people financially. Unemployed people with AIDS or ARC have few options. They often cannot find more work and thus another group health insurance plan. Some try and move in with someone who can add them to their own job-related health insurance. Often they end up spending their life savings in a short period of time and seeking public assistance. Because of lack of money, they often have to leave their dwellings and seek a less expensive living space. A sudden loss of insurance necessitates drastic adjustments at a time when AIDS or ARC patients can least afford it. In rare cases companies continue to pay for the insurance of AIDS or ARC patients after they cannot work. The authors would like to commend this kind of behavior as a humane short-term solution to what is a gigantic and growing dilemma—how to insure AIDS-virus-positive individuals.

The question of how to distribute the risk of insuring infected individuals may cause a major crisis in the insurance industry. Insurance in general is based on the notion of defined risk. Individuals buy insurance because they feel the cost to them is worth protecting the losses they would incur if certain events, such as fire, car accident, or disabling disease, were to take place. Insurance companies operate on the principle that they can reliably define the risks against which they insure. Rates are set so that over a large population and a long period of time companies will be able to provide the coverage, pay the claims they insure against and still realize a profit.

Insurance companies do not like to insure an undefinable risk. Since the long-term medical prognosis for AIDS-virus-positive people is so unclear, the idea of having more than 1 million infected Americans is frightening indeed to the insurance industry. With the natural history of AIDS virus a long way from being described, what are reasonable policies to account for this unknown risk?

In the first half of 1985, laws were passed in both Wisconsin and California that make it illegal for insurers or employers to use a positive result on the AIDS virus blood test as a basis for denying employment or insurance. (This protects symptomless carriers of the AIDS virus but not individuals who have been treated for AIDS or ARC.) Both statutes were carefully shepherded through the respective state legislatures. No public hearings were held and the statutes were attached to bills that were virtually assured of passing. They may have been more of a testament to political skill than a measurement of public consensus.

Insurance companies fear that large numbers of infected individuals will purchase large amounts of life insurance, health insurance, and disability insurance and at the same rates as uninfected individuals. These fears are fueled by reports of large payments in life insurance claims of AIDS patients. General Reassurance Corporation has found the amount on all AIDS life insurance claims typically five times the average. In certain populations, notably gay males in San Francisco, it is estimated that 70% or more are already infected with the virus. If it turns out that these individuals have a dramatically shortened life expectancy, and if many of these individuals buy large amounts of life insurance, companies may be paying tens or even hundreds of millions of dollars in life insurance claims as well as millions more in disability and medical claims.

It is obvious that a scenario such as the one above could not continue indefinitely. At some point an insurance company would have to either be allowed to identify these higher risk individuals (through blood testing) or else distribute the risk some other way. It is likely that remedial legislation will be sought that will permit blood testing for the AIDS virus by insurance companies. One approach is to deny coverage to people believed to be at higher risk than normal. A medical record that includes a history of sexually transmitted disease might cause insurance companies to take a second look at an application. Another "red flag" is a large individual policy (life, health, or disability) by a person with little "insurable interest" (property, high income, ownership of a business).

Another approach would be to redistribute risk according to categories that correlate with AIDS cases. Rates might be raised according to age, marital status, or proximity to an area of high prevalence of AIDS virus infection. This means that uninfected individuals in these categories would pay increased premiums. With tens of billions of dollars in hospitalization expenses for the AIDS patients of the next few years, the insurance issue is crucial. It can be safely said that this issue is going to be determined as the natural history of AIDS virus infection becomes further defined. The worse the long-term medical prognosis for infected individuals, the stronger would be the argument for classification on the basis of infection.

There is an interrelationship between insurability and employability. If a potential employee is infected with the AIDS virus, he or she represents an influence that may eventually lead to higher group rates for an employer. In April 1985 the city of Hollywood, Florida, announced that it planned to use the AIDS virus blood test to screen applicants. The reason cited was a desire to avoid an adverse impact on health insurance rates. According to Charlotte Crenson, spokesperson for Blue Cross–Blue Shield, this is not unrealistic. She stated that a number of AIDS cases in a company's work force could increase its premiums for medical benefits.

As of late August 1985, Wisconsin and California are the

only states that prohibit the use of the AIDS virus blood test to determine insurability. Many companies are in the process of developing policies to deal with this troubling issue. Even if decisions were made to include a blood test as part of an insurance application, it would take several months for a company to gear up for its use. What actions will insurance companies take for AIDS-virus-positive people? They may greatly increase their rates, or they may find a justification for refusing to insure them.

It is clear that with the current growth in infection in combination with an ambiguous medical future for the infected, the AIDS epidemic may force a major readjustment by the insurance industry. Insurance is considered so vital by those who work with AIDS victims because it pays the medical bills. But in view of staggering increases in AIDS-related health care costs, the growing question is: How will the bills be paid?

Paying the Bill

By the end of 1985 there will be at least 1.5 million Americans infected with the AIDS virus. This means that 150,000 AIDS cases will appear by the end of 1988. At the International Conference on AIDS in Atlanta in April 1985, Dr. Ann Hardy, director of public health for the Centers for Disease Control, estimated that each AIDS patient costs $140,000 in hospitalization expenses. This figure may *increase* in the future due to the development of therapies that will prolong life but not restore health. If this is true, the hospitalization expense for AIDS patients who are already "on their way" is $21 billion. The expense for ARC patients, larger in number but smaller in average expense, should add several billion more.

It is important to emphasize that this "bill" is inevitable. Every day, as new people are infected the amount grows. If the conservative projection of 1,000 new people infected each day is correct, then we can expect 100 new AIDS cases to develop from those infections, for a daily "bill" of $14 million. If the more dramatic figures of Dr. Bolognesi are used, the daily bill soars to $70 million.

These figures only estimate the amount of direct financial outlays to pay for the hospitalization of these patients. There is a greater loss to our society in terms of lost future earnings due to disability and premature death. Dr. Hardy calculated that an average of more than $600,000 per patient would be lost in future earnings. This means that our nation will lose $75 billion in earnings from the first 150,000 AIDS patients. The AIDS epidemic has already cost our society at least $100 billion.

It is in light of calculations such as these that the current 1986 federal budget projection of $196 million must be analyzed. The federal government intends to devote $196 million to a problem that already has "created a bill" of at least $100 billion.

The Subcommittee on Health and the Environment, chaired by Congressman Henry Waxman of California, was instrumental in encouraging a budget increase of nearly 100% devoted to AIDS in fiscal year 1986. The Department of Health and Human Services is also to be commended for responding, if belatedly, to this pressing need. A budget increase of nearly 100% is impressive at a time when fiscal restraint is a widely promoted value. Many of the research projects in the revised budget proposal are important areas for investigation. However, it is quite clear that AIDS requires a much larger response. How much money should be allocated for AIDS research? Even an unlimited amount of funding might not lead to a solution. There is a limit to how much can be profitably spent without redirecting current research projects which are also important to the national interest.

The "AIDS bill" will be paid from three sources—individual wealth, the insurance industry, and taxation. Currently, there is no coherent plan to pay for the medical expenses of patients with AIDS. Individuals are left to fend for themselves, making out the best they can with a combination of personal savings, insurance, family contributions, and public assistance. Will some sort of "formula" evolve that takes into account an individual's financial situation (much like the system for aid at many colleges)?

Recent national attention has shown that people, when asked in a public opinion poll, indicate willingness to have their taxes raised to pay for AIDS research. However, with the current bill at $21 billion, and with experts predicting a doubling of infection each year for the rest of the decade, there will come a point when some troubling questions such as the following will be raised.

Why should monogamous people be taxed to pay for a disease that is transmitted through sexual contact? There will no doubt continue to be many more urban AIDS cases than rural AIDS cases. Will rural people be willing to be taxed to pay for a disease that is so prevalent in cities? AIDS cases will undoubtedly occur in far greater numbers of unmarried people than married poeple. Will married people be willing to be taxed to pay for the unfortunate results of promiscuous activities of unmarried people? The greatest number of cases, nearly half, will continue to be diagnosed in people 35 years old or younger. Will middle-aged and older people be willing to be taxed to pay for a disease of the young?

The battle for how research money should be allocated is also fraught with political implications. Advocates of high-risk groups (of which the gays are the most politically well organized) push for massive funding on research for treatment for AIDS. Others feel that a larger public good could be served by the development of a vaccination, which could prevent the spread of the virus to the large percentage of uninfected Americans. In a recent poll 56% of the people listed the development of a vaccine as the top research priority. Research on a cure was listed as the top concern of 28% of the respondents. It would not be surprising to see a funding battle between those who desire more research and others who feel funds should be allocated to restrict the freedoms of infected people.

The AIDS epidemic is an evolving national emergency.

There exist a multitude of competing interests, each with legitimate concerns. Health care professionals who serve AIDS patients would like more research done on possible cures. Many of them are aware that there are tens of thousands of AIDS patients who will be appearing in the next few years. The health care system will have to make a major adjustment. Today's resources are inadequate to meet this onslaught. There is no system to pay for the hospitalization expenses of these unfortunate individuals.

A related problem is to find enough health care workers willing and emotionally able to treat these people. Working on the AIDS ward is the least desirable alternative to many people in the field. The fear of infection and the depressing aspect of seeing so many young dying people make volunteers less than plentiful. Already there are signs of "burnout." In addition to primary patient care, there must be support services to cope with the psychosocial needs of AIDS patients and their loved ones.

Epidemiologists are concerned about slowing the spread of infection. Every day that 1,000 or more people are infected, the size of our national problem grows larger. And, of course, every infected person appears to be permanently infectious and the large percentage are unaware of their infection. We don't really know how many are infected or how quickly the virus is spreading. Massive education appears to be the only hope, as restrictive measures would be for the most part ineffective or impossible to implement. How can the spread of infection be stopped?

The insurance industry is in a quandary. This epidemic is costly and was unanticipated. It does not show signs of receding, at least in the next several years. Since the natural history of AIDS virus infection is defined in an ambiguous way, for a short (five-year) period of time the construction of reasonable actuarial tables will continue to be impossible. Insurance companies have obligations to those already insured to provide reasonable coverage. There are also obligations to the general public to provide a mechanism for guarding against future financial catastrophe, as well as to employees and stockholders to maintain profitability. What are rational policies, both short and long term, by which the insurance industry can properly meet its obligations?

There are over 1 million infected Americans. Their rights must be protected. AIDS virus infection should not resign an individual to second-class citizenship. But these rights must be protected in a way that also protects the public health. There are (hopefully) small numbers of infected individuals who exhibit reckless disregard for the rights of others by unwillingly exposing others to infection. There should be a mechanism to prevent and punish this type of behavior. How can a balance be struck between the protection of individual rights and protection of the public health?

All sides in this crisis will eventually have to compromise if there is to be a coherent national response. Work must proceed on possible treatments and a vaccine. The spread of the virus must be slowed. The expenses of AIDS patients must be anticipated. The rights of both infected and uninfected individuals must be protected.

Every American will eventually pay a price for the AIDS epidemic. The price will include increased taxes, increased insurance rates, and some degree of lost freedom. The population most affected by AIDS is at the peak of their earning power. Without their energy, productivity, and consumption, the economy will be crippled, resulting in declining business conditions and an eroding tax base. In addition, there will be an eventual loss of leadership, managerial, and creative talent certainly equivalent to that lost in a major war. Our nation must respond effectively, coherently, and immediately.

We believe that if our nation continues to react to the AIDS epidemic in convulsive lurches we are doomed to an extraordinarily grim future. We strongly favor the immediate convening of a Presidential "blue ribbon panel" to recommend policies for both the short and long term which will help our nation respond to this mess. This group should include distinguished members representing a variety of concerns—epidemiologists, physicians, research scientists, the insurance industry, civil-liberties advocates, and informed citizens. Until representatives of the competing interests in this dilemma begin to develop cooperative approaches, our nation will continue to be unpleasantly surprised by the enormity and complexity of this growing epidemic.

CHAPTER 9 REFERENCES

1. Experience with HTLV-III Antibody Testing–Update On: Screening and Epidemiology, Sponsored by the Center for Drugs and Biology, Food and Drug Administration, National Institutes of Health, and the Centers for Disease Control, July 31, 1985.

2. Filson CR, Tartaglia CR, Tello MA, at al. Psychological Concerns of Individuals with AIDS Related Concerns (abst). International Conference on Acquired Immune Deficiency Syndrome (AIDS). Atlanta, GA, April 14-17, 1985, p. 66.

3. Bruno GG. The Psychosocial Effects of AIDS Related Complex (ARC) on Young Adult Hemophiliacs (abst). International Conference on Acquired Immune Deficiency Syndrome (AIDS). Atlanta, GA, April 14-17, 1985, p. 66.

4. Christ GH, and Wiener CS. Psychosocial Issues and AIDS. In *AIDS: Etiology, Diagnosis, Treatment, and Prevention.* DeVita VT, Hellman S, Rosenbert SA (eds) J.B. Lippincott Company, New York, p. 275, 1985.

5. Wilson MB, Surmall K, Scott WA, et al. AIDS Prevention: A Three Year/Three Phase Approach (abst). International Conference on Acquired Immune Deficiency Syndrome (AIDS). Atlanta, GA, April 14-17, 1985, p. 61.

6. Bross DC. Legal aspects of STD control. In *Sexually Transmitted Diseases.* Holmes KK, Mardl P, Sparling PF, Wiesner PJ (eds). McGraw-Hill Book Company, New York, p. 925-930, 1984.

10

Passing the Torch

Today our nation is in the midst of the greatest public health crisis of the twentieth century. Less than 10 years since it first came to these shores, the AIDS virus has infected more than 1 million Americans. During the past few years, there has been an incredible explosion of infection with the AIDS virus. In early 1982 less than 100,000 Americans were infected with the virus. By early 1986 more than 1.5 million Americans will be infected.

What is worse, more than 90% of those who are infected do not know it. A fatal, sexually transmitted germ that creates no immediate signs is an epidemiologist's nightmare. That is precisely what is running loose in the sexually active circles in our society.

Although medical science is investigating possible treatments or vaccines, to suggest that one is imminent would be criminal. Public health officials feel that the development of a vaccine or treatment will probably not occur until at least 1990. Many feel that this prediction is too optimistic.

AIDS has already ravaged urban, gay America. In some cities, more than three-fourths of the sexually active men have the virus. The presence of the AIDS virus in heterosexual circles in our country is a certainty. Once the virus achieves a "portal of entry" into a promiscuous population, it spreads quickly. Without widely available blood testing, we do not know the prevalence of the virus in populations not currently defined as being high risk.

The AIDS virus spread through Africa the same way that herpes spread throughout America—through a promiscuous, heterosexual population. As soon as the AIDS virus achieves a "foothold" in promiscuous heterosexual circles, the prevalence of infection will again be explosive. Like the second-stage rocket booster, this may put AIDS virus infection "into orbit." It is not out of the question that without some serious, immediate steps, 10 to 30 million Americans may be infected by the end of this decade.

What would it mean to our society to have 10 million people, most of them young, infected with the AIDS virus by 1990? Without some currently unexpected medical miracle, what would the future hold for these people? It is expected that between 500,000 and 1 million people would die as the result of AIDS within five years. An additional 2.5 million would experience the medical signs and symptoms of AIDS-related complex (ARC). None of them should marry, bear natural children, or have normal sexual relations.

The financial burden alone that would be created almost defies imagination: It currently costs $140,000 to treat each AIDS patient. The medical bill for 1 million AIDS patients would exceed $100 billion. When adding to this the wages lost due to disability and premature death, the bill comes to nearly three quarters of a trillion dollars, or one-fourth of our current gross national product! These are not imaginary numbers. They are frighteningly real.

The AIDS virus may turn our society into something none of us would like. A society with hundreds of thousands or millions of sick and dying young people is one with its lifeblood drained. A society that, for the public good, restricts choices in career, marriage, and childbearing is a society of greatly reduced freedom, closed frontiers, and limited options. A society in which millions of citizens wake up each day fearing a slight fever or swollen glands is a society of dread and depression.

It is no wonder that at a July 1985 Congressional hearing, Dr. Michael Gottlieb, an immunologist at UCLA, said, "The long-term consequences of this epidemic are as significant as drought or famine. It will continue to erode the resources of this nation if we do not respond effectively."

If we are to mount a response appropriate to the size of the threat, we must first rid ourselves of the cherished bromides that temporarily comfort some at the price of long-term destruction. Vague, unfocused hope, vindictiveness, smallmindedness, and prejudice will not get the job done. Here are three "non-solutions" that must be abandoned.

Fixing the Blame

There exists a band of zealots dedicated to using the AIDS crisis as a political platform for their narrow points of view. According to them, homosexuals are "sinners in the hands of an angry God" who are receiving their just punishment. It is hard to summon breath to respond to this notion, which is not only untrue and cruel but counterproductive.

Homosexuals are not responsible for the existence of the AIDS virus. They were not the agents that brought the virus to the Western Hemisphere. The urban, male, homosexual community first felt the brunt of the burden that AIDS has begun to create. It has already experienced a tremendous amount of death and sickness due to AIDS, and it has produced the first models of community support for the victims of this tragic disease.

The subject of "blame" should not be a part of the public debate about AIDS, and it certainly is not part of the solution. Had God intended to "punish" homosexuals, why were homosexual females excluded? Why were hemophiliacs and blood transfusion recipients included in this curiously selective "scourge"? What possible divine motive could there be for the death of infants due to AIDS?

Unfortunate victims of the AIDS virus, past, present, and future, will have had enough pain and agony without having to add blame to the list. All the attention focused on "blaming" is wasted energy. Vicious individuals who continue to use the AIDS crisis for their own personal and political vendettas should be hooted off the stage of public debate. They contribute nothing.

Ignoring and Understating the Threat

Just as there exists a core of people who use the AIDS crisis to merchandise their biblical, apocalyptic vision, there also exists a group that is dedicated to preaching "moderation" in the name of preserving public sanity. Moderate, soothing, comforting words are not the order of the day. Warning of the dangers posed by the AIDS virus should be shouted for all to hear.

Unfortunately, in this group of "caution merchants" there are individuals so close to the problem that they should know better. Spokespersons for the Centers for Disease Control in particular have seemed reluctant to identify heterosexual spread of the AIDS virus as the threat it undoubtedly represents. The CDC method of categorizing AIDS patients so as to minimize the number reported due to "heterosexual spread" allows heterosexuals to feel an improper sense of security.

The desire not to be a bearer of bad news or appear to be an "alarmist" is understandable. But it is impossible to understand why it is more important to prevent anxiety than to prevent death. By 1990 millions of heterosexuals will be infected with the AIDS virus. It is hard to imagine that any of them would be willing to trade a life of solitude, restriction, fear, and uncertainty for a few years of "fun." Cushioning the truth endorses heterosexual spread.

There should be no leeway in public pronouncements of responsible officials. AIDS is a deadly threat. The virus victimizes all whom it infects. It is sexually transmitted, and undoubtedly it has gained a "foothold" in the heterosexual population. It can be correctly stated that an ounce of prevention is worth a ton of cure.

As part of this trend of "moderation," there is ambiguity in the terminology used in discussing AIDS. Many spokespersons are unwilling to use the term "infected" when referring to someone who has been infected with the AIDS virus. The word "exposed," more palatable and ambiguous, is frequently substituted.

At the July 31, 1985, meeting at the National Institutes of Health to discuss results of the first four months of national screening for the AIDS virus, one doctor, an official of the American Red Cross, was questioned on this point. He was asked if donors with a repeatedly positive ELISA result (confirmed by Western blot analysis) were informed that they had been "exposed to" or "infected by" the AIDS virus. Although evidence for use of the word "infected" is conclusive, the official declined to answer the question directly. He referred it to another member of the Red Cross, who waffled, saying, "Generally, they are told that they *may have been exposed*, or that *there is a likelihood that they may have been exposed* and that they may be infectious." (Emphasis supplied.)

Another favorite semantic game played by advocates of "moderation" is the claim that "we do not really know the significance of seropositivity" (i.e., a positive blood test for the AIDS virus). That is also ridiculous. If the blood test is performed rigorously, and if an initial positive outcome is confirmed by another test (e.g., the Western blot), we *do* know the significance of seropositivity. In 999 out of 1,000 cases, it means that the individual has been infected with the AIDS virus! Infected individuals should consider themselves to be infectious for an undetermined amount of time; they should refrain from sex, postpone marriage, and not bear children. Furthermore, they might suffer potential employment and insurance consequences, and they may at any time, without warning, develop AIDS or ARC.

The examples above illustrate the ambiguous terminology employed by "merchants of caution." Although there is some value in trying to assuage the emotions of infected individuals, such terms allow the general public to continue to underestimate the threat of AIDS.

Underplaying the threat is close to encouraging the spread of the virus. Ignoring the threat is worse. AIDS presents to our society the first infectious, deadly disease that kills young people since the polio epidemic. Perhaps it is due to this that people seem to be reluctant to confront it until it "shows up on the doorstep." If you do not believe this is true, then try to talk with someone intelligently about AIDS for more than a few minutes. It is so unpleasant that people invariably find "something to do."

AIDS is, unfortunately, here to stay. It challenges our national resourcefulness. Closing our eyes and opening them in the hope that AIDS will somehow disappear will not help; it will only allow matters to worsen.

Hoping That "They Figure Out What to Do"

Medical science is doing the best that can be done with the time and resources available. Even if researchers had an unlimited amount of funding, the solution to the AIDS problem will not be developed quickly. The nature of retroviruses, of which the AIDS is one, makes them an especially vexing medical problem. Because they genetically "interpose" themselves within the cells of the invaded host, retroviruses have so far proven to be impossible to kill. The medical problems that they present will not be solved overnight, and in fact, if any answer is developed within a decade, it will be a very significant accomplishment.

The hope that government, or scientific research, will come up with a "solution" to AIDS is somewhat understandable. Less than a decade ago, inflation and oil dependence seemed to be insurmountable problems. Now on public opinion polls, they are rarely listed among the top concerns.

To abdicate a personal sense of responsibility to the hope that a medical miracle will render this concern obsolete is reckless and naive. In fact, this problem requires a focusing of national will that is unlike anything observed since World War II. The need for individual and civic responsibility has never been more paramount. If AIDS does have a solution, it is in the individual that the answer resides—expressing concern, educating others, mobilizing political support, and most of all, taking responsibility for sexual choices. What can be done? There are a number of things an individual can do to be mobilized against the AIDS virus.

Recognize and Accept the Magnitude of the Threat

Counselors say that the most important step someone can take in combating a problem such as alcohol or drug abuse is to utter the magic four-word phrase, "I have a problem." What is true for individuals is also true for a society. When the day comes that our nation finally takes a deep, collective breath, looks at AIDS, and concludes that "we have a problem" is the day we start on the road to a solution.

Denial of reality does not change anything—it makes everything worse. Do not permit yourself the luxury of wishful thinking about AIDS. Do not be placated or distracted by the "merchants of caution." Some of them appear to be pursuing political agendas rather than contributing wholeheartedly to solving the problem. Do not allow demagogues to frame the issues; there is plenty of real work to be done and self-appointed moral referees will only get in the way.

AIDS is not a homosexual disease. A cure or vaccination is not imminent. The problem is much larger than those who have contracted the end-stage disease. All infected people, who now number more than a million, are victims even when they are symptomless.

Educate Others—Contribute to the Public Dialogue

In addition to recognizing these truths, you can make a great contribution by conveying them to others. The issue of AIDS must become a matter of public discussion. Do not allow prejudice to control the agenda. Ignorance and complacency are two of the greatest allies of the AIDS virus. They create a climate in which the virus can thrive.

Frank discussion of these facts is necessary in order to marshal a coherent response to the threat of AIDS. Discussions of them will not be cheerful, friendly conversations, but they may save lives. An immediate, realizable goal is to see to it that no Americans are comfortable with the rationalizations that up to this point have substituted for factual public discourse about AIDS. There is no time to luxuriate in our prejudices. The development of a rational public dialogue about AIDS is a beginning.

It is, however, only a beginning. AIDS is not only a medical crisis but a crisis of national resources, civil liberties, and basic questions about the freedom to choose. The AIDS crisis will cause Americans to examine their values in order to answer questions such as these: What restrictions, if any, should be placed on infected people to help slow the spread of a potentially fatal disease? Should government be allowed to decide who can or cannot bear children? If government will ultimately pay the bill, what steps are justifiable in order to prevent further spread of AIDS virus infection? What insurance consequences should arise from a positive blood test for the virus? Do infected people have the same "rights" as uninfected people in buying insurance? Why should monogamous, uninfected people pay higher rates in order to pay claims resulting from a sexually transmitted disease? What information about this disease should be distributed? Which is more important—protecting the rights of infected individuals or the lives of uninfected individuals?

This is just a sample of the questions that will spring out of this crisis. By forcing discussion of the AIDS problem, you will contribute to slowing the spread, which means that you will save lives. It is an interesting paradox that the more "alarmist" the discussion now, the less drastic will be the measures that may be necessary during the future. The specter of 10 or 20 million infected people in the United States and the lack of an effective cure might necessitate drastic government action. Voluntary prevention of spread is by far preferable to involuntary, restrictive measures that may be inevitable if the involuntary actions do not work.

One part of the campaign of nationally disseminating information about AIDS should be carried out in public schools. Although there is a great deal that is not yet understood about AIDS, such as the long-term natural history of the disease, there is a certain amount that we do understand. We can say with confidence that AIDS is caused by a virus that can be transmitted sexually and through the blood. Fortunately, AIDS has not affected significant numbers of teenagers. By making high school students aware of some basic information about AIDS, such as how it is transmitted, we may be able to provide an "emotional inoculation" of sorts.

Have Your Blood Tested and Encourage Others to Do So

While research on a cure continues as rapidly as is possible, a great deal of attention should be given to preventing the spread of the virus. Beyond educating people as to the true nature of the problem, there is no more important priority than making the AIDS virus blood test available and "consequence free." Since most infected individuals do not realize that they are infected and infectious, the

AIDS virus continues to spread under this "cloak of invisibility." Its prevalence in the heterosexual community is simply not known.

There are numerous problems inherent in identifying the infected individuals. First, it must be logistically possible to perform the large number of blood tests that the present dilemma warrants. This means that there must be a massive "gearing up" of laboratories that can perform both the simple ELISA tests and the more difficult Western blot test. Fortunately, most ELISA tests will be negative, which will make it unnecessary to do Western blot analysis. However, it is currently difficult to process accurately all donated blood. Because of the possibility of "false negatives" (infected blood that does not show up as being infected), the Red Cross does not want people to use blood donations as a "surrogate AIDS virus test." For these reasons, in most communities it is possible to have the blood test done confidentially at a separate facility. However, only those in the high-risk groups with strong reason to suspect infection are encouraged to take the test. In light of limited facilities, it is understandable to try to limit the number of tests run. However, as the result of this policy, it is difficult for those who may be now infecting others to find out whether or not they are infected.

Making the blood test available on a confidential basis to all who wish to be tested should be an immediate national policy objective. To accomplish this, two actions are necessary: First, the money should be allocated to allow for extensive testing on a local or regional basis. Second, the federal government and the insurance industry should reach some sort of agreement so that a "truce" or period of moratorium can be declared. Eventually, the AIDS virus blood test sequence will probably be part of insurance-application processes. However, in the interest of preventing the spread (certainly in the long-term interest of the industry itself), a moratorium of, say, one year should be declared. During this period, the insurance companies should be unable to use the blood test to determine rates or insurability. This would protect the insurance rights of the symptomless carriers—that is, by far the majority of infected individuals. ARC and AIDS patients would suffer insurance consequences as a result of medical documentation of their conditions. Blood testing of the AIDS virus can be done confidentially by assigning a number to those who wish the test to be run and informing them of the result according to that number.

One of the major expenses in taking this drastic but necessary step will be the cost of providing counseling services to those who have a positive result on the blood test. This, too, takes money. But the step of making the AIDS virus blood test available and "consequence free" is the most productive, rational, cost-effective way of slowing the spread of infections.

How can an individual affect this process? First of all, start by calling your local public health department and ask where you can get the AIDS virus blood test. At some point you will be asked to give the reason for your request. If you are not a member of a currently identified high-risk group (male homosexuals, recent immigrants from Haiti or central Africa, hemophiliacs, intravenous drug abusers, and the sexual partners of anyone in a high-risk group), you may be either strongly discouraged from taking the test or told that you cannot take it.

One factor that will be mentioned is the possibility of "false positive" outcomes. Remember, this is to a great extent a bluff. False positives occur on the initial ELISA test. When the entire sequence is run (including the Western blot test), there are very few false positives. Find out from the person with whom you speak when blood tests will be readily available. Talk to someone in a position of authority. Create pressure at the local level for this necessary action. Write your governmental representatives in your state capital and in Washington, D.C. Make this a vital, urgent issue! Until this step is accomplished, the AIDS virus will have "free run." The longer we wait to make the test available to everyone, the more serious the problem will become.

Prevent the Sexual Spread

By far most infections with the AIDS virus will occur as a result of sexual transmission. The problems associated with preventing the sexual transmission of the AIDS virus are well documented. Since the AIDS virus does not cause any obvious signs or symptoms soon after it has infected an individual, most infected individuals remain unaware of their infection for a considerable period of time after they have been infected. Thus a few promiscuous, infected individuals who are unaware of their infection with the virus can cause a great number of infections during a short period of time. This has been demonstrated by the fact that the AIDS virus has infected a considerable percentage of sexually active members of certain populations.

Gay activists have pointed to certain statements that indicate fear of heterosexual spread of the virus as being prejudicial against gays. For example, in an address at the International Conference on AIDS in Atlanta during April 1985, Margaret Heckler (Secretary for Health and Human Services) said, "We must stop this before it gets out into the general population."

The infection of a homosexual man is no less cause for concern than the infection of a heterosexual man or woman. The reason for the concern about heterosexual spread is simply this: With roughly 20 times as many heterosexual men and women as there are homosexual men, the AIDS virus can quickly infect millions of people. The possibility that the AIDS virus will make a quantum jump in the numbers it infects is cause for serious concern. There is a vast difference, for example, between 2 million and 20 million.

How can the heterosexual spread of the AIDS virus be moderated? Certainly, the widespread availability of "consequence free" blood testing will make a large difference, but to wait for that step would be waiting too long. Heterosexuals must make some serious, pragmatic revisions in their sexual habits. Each new partner is a potential source of infection. Epidemiological analyses suggest that there is a correlation between the development of AIDS and promiscuity. However, this is not due to having had sex with "too many" partners. It is more due to having had sex with the "wrong partner."

There are two ways to slow the sexual spread of the AIDS virus: reduce the number of new partners, and reduce the possibility of infection through the practice of "safe sex."

Will heterosexual Americans acquire a "new morality"? If so, this will be a morality based on pragmatism rather than on scriptural advice. If the AIDS virus spreads among heterosexual Americans and begins to victimize people, there will certainly be an evolution to this lifestyle, as there has been in many homosexual circles. Will this result from anticipation of the spread of the virus or will it be a reaction to its spread?

Alert Your Representatives

The threat represented by the AIDS virus requires responses at all levels of government. In some senses the heterosexual spread of the virus, which will create national "shock waves," may mobilize the national consensus, thus eventually leading to benefits for both "gay" and "straight" Americans.

On a local level, school administrations should be made aware of the necessity for doing at least some basic introductory teaching about AIDS as part of the standard health education curriculum. With regard to funding for AIDS research, Dr. Paul Volberding of San Francisco General Hospital recently said at a July 1985 Congressional hearing, "In addition to an AIDS vaccine, we need to support a much more *vigorous program of public education.* While AIDS is a complex disease, its transmission is well understood and preventable." (Emphasis supplied.)

State governments could contribute to slowing the

spread of the AIDS virus by disseminating information through state universities. Certainly, a synopsis of the threat of the end stages of the disease, the ambiguities about the development of the disease, and the means of preventing the spread (e.g., blood tests, reduction of the number of sexual partners and the practice of "safe sex") could be put into easily distributed pamphlets. This would at least be a start.

The federal government is, obviously, going to be caught in a "crossfire." The Reagan administration has asked Congress to boost research funds by more than 100%, a considerable figure for these days of budget cuts. It is recommending that there be $196.3 million in the 1986 budget for AIDS. This amount, however, is a "drop in the bucket" when considering the size of the problem. In assessing the amount of money that should be allocated, the federal government should consider not only how best to respond to the present situation but also how to prevent the situation from becoming impossibly expensive during the future.

The federal government has another important role. It must become a leader in stepping into this "snake pit" of confusing priorities and contradictory questions and in defining some terms. A "blue ribbon panel" would not necessarily *solve* these problems, but it could provide a forum for communication and compromise. Until we resolve the "Gordian knot" of insurance and civil liberties issues, at least for some time there will be little hope of significantly slowing the spread of infection.

The longer our society delays its response to the spread of the virus, the more severe the consequences will be. There will be more people infected, more lives lost, more careers interrupted, and more fear spread. The government will respond appropriately when individuals mobilize and express their concern. By contacting your elected local, state, and federal officials, you can take a small but helpful stand in the interest of all.

*   *   *

How will our nation respond to this epidemic—the greatest threat to the public health in our history? In the past, Americans have reasserted their national strength during crises. AIDS may lead to a national hysteria of selfishness or a national revolution of brotherhood and heroism. The AIDS crisis may divide our nation, or it may unite it.

The most quintessential part of the American dream is to be able to leave future generations a better life. On January 20, 1961, President John F. Kennedy said, "Let the word go forth from this time and place…that the torch has been passed to a new generation of Americans." President Theodore Roosevelt wrote of this concept a few months before his death. He had heard of the death of his youngest son, Quentin, killed in combat during World War I. He wrote, "In America today all our people are summoned to service and sacrifice…But all of us who give service, and stand ready for sacrifice, are the torch-bearers. We run with the torches until we fall, content if we can then pass them on to the hands of other runners."

The AIDS epidemic could be the greatest challenge presented to civilization during this century. The AIDS virus is a foe fully as dangerous as any military force ever assembled. To presume that some brilliant scientist will miraculously absolve us of our individual and civic responsibilities is to mortgage the future to a mere hope.

How will we respond? What kind of world will we leave our children? How will we do at carrying our generation's torch? We are at a fork in the road. The time to respond is now.

APPENDIX A

A Partial List of Organizations Involved in AIDS Lobbying, Public Education, Prevention, or Social Services

EAST COAST

GLH/AIDS Project
P.O. Box 11013
Durham, NC
(919) 286-0079

Gay Men's Alliance of
   Hudson Valley
255 Grove St.
White Plains, NY 10601
(914) 997-5149

Long Island AIDS Project
SUNY Health Sciences
Stony Brook, NY 11794
(516) 444-2403

AIDS Task Force, Inc.
P.O. Box 3B/Bidwell
Buffalo, NY 14222
(716) 886-1275

AIDS Program, HCC, Inc.
50 Court St., Suite 1001
Brooklyn, NY 11201
(212) 855-7275

SouTier AIDS Task Force
P.O. Box 1492
Binghampton, NY 13902
(607) 723-6493

Central NY AIDS Task
   Force
P.O. Box 1682
Syracuse, NY 13201
(315) 475-2430

AIDS Rochester, Inc.
153 Liberty Poleway
Rochester, NY 14604
(716) 232-7181

Capitol District AIDS
332 Hudson Ave.
Albany, NY 12110
(518) 465-6094

Haitian Coalition on AIDS
255 Eastern Parkway
Brooklyn, NY 11238
(212) 783-2676

AIDS Task Force
CDGLF, Box 131
Albany, NY 12201
(518) 465-6094

Lambda Legal Defense and
   Education Fund
132 W. 43rd St.
New York, NY 10036
(212) 944-9488

Haitian Committee on
AIDS
117 Harvard St.
Dorchester, MA 02124
(617) 436-2808

Fenway Health Community
   Center/AIDS Action
   Committee
16 Haviland St.
Boston, MA 02115
(617) 267-7573

Gay Men's Health Crisis,
   Inc.
Box 274, 132 W. 24th St.
New York, NY 10011
(212) 807-6664

AID Atlanta
1132 W. Peachtree, NW, #112
Atlanta, GA 30309
(408) 872-0600

Philadelphia AIDS Task
   Force
P.O. Box 7259
Philadelphia, PA 19101
(215) 232-8055

AIDS Educ. Program
5900 W. Junior Coll. Rd.
Key West, FL 33040

AIDS Education Fund
2335 18th St.,
N.W.Washington, D.C.
20009
(202) 332-5939

AIDS Project New Haven
P.O. Box 7
New Haven, CT 06473
(203) 239-7881

Gay and Lesbian Alliance
   of Delaware
P.O. Box 9218
Wilmington, DE 19809
(302) 764-2208

AIDS Action Committee
P.O. Box 4073
Key West, FL 33041
(305) 294-5531, ext. 4797

Health Crisis Net.
1930 Bay Drive, #2
Normandy Isle, FL 33141
(305) 448-2882

HERO/Medical Arts Bldg.
Cathedral & Read, #819
Baltimore, MD 21201
(301) 955-3150

Gay Rights National Lobby
   AIDS Project
P.O. Box 1892
Washington, D.C. 20013
(202) 546-1801

The Bar Association for
   Human Rights for
   Greater New York
P.O. Box 1899
Grand Central Station
New York, NY 10163

United States Conference of Mayors
1620 I St., N.W.
Washington, D.C.
(202) 254-8718

National Gay Task Force
80 Fifth Ave.
New York, NY 10011
(212) 714-5800

AIDS Action Council
Federation of AIDS-Related
  Organizations
1115½ Independence Ave.,
  S.E.
Washington, D.C. 20003
(202) 547-3101/547-3102

Mayor's Interagency Task
  Force on AIDS
1025 Worth St., Rm. 604
New York, NY 10013
(212) 566-0484

AIDS Resource Center, Inc.
235 W. 18th St.
New York, NY 10011
(212) 206-1414

AIDS Medical Foundation
230 Park Ave., Rm. 1266
New York, NY 10169
(212) 949-7410

AIDS Network Group
Department of Social Work
Memorial Sloan-Kettering
1275 York Ave.
New York, NY 10021
(212) 794-7018

Haitian Community Health
  Project
391 Eastern Parkway
Brooklyn, NY 11213
(718) 773-1171

AIDS Institute
New York State Department
  of Health
8 E. 40th St., 3rd floor
New York, NY 10016
(212) 340-3388

Lesbian and Gay Concern
  Committee
  National Association of
  Social Workers
110 W. 86th St.
New York, NY 10024
(212) 799-3298

West Coast

AIDS Team
P.O. Box 9773
Fresno, CA 93974
(209) 264-2436

Pacific Center AIDS Project
2712 Telegraph Ave.
Berkeley, CA 94705
(415) 548-8283

AIDS Education/Research
  Foundation
P.O. Box 14227
San Francisco, CA 94123
(415) 626-8784

SF People with AIDS
1040 Ashbury, #5
San Francisco, CA 94117
(415) 665-3787

Los Angeles AIDS Network
811 N. Coronado Terrace
Los Angeles, CA 90026
(213) 483-8574

AIDS InterFaith Network
890 Hayes St.
San Francisco, CA 94117
(415) 558-9644

American Association of
  Physicians for Human
  Rights
P.O. Box 14546
San Francisco, CA 94114
(415) 673-3189

Seattle AIDS Action Comm.
113 Summit Ave. E., #204
Seattle, WA 98104
(206) 323-1229

Northwest AIDS
  Foundation
P.O. Box 3449
Seattle, WA 98114
(206) 527-8770; 622-9650;
  322-6698

Gay Men's Health Group
2353 Minor Ave. E.
Seattle, WA 98102
(206) 322-3919

Seattle Gay Clinic
P.O. Box 20066
Seattle, WA 98104
(206) 322-2873

Cascade AIDS Project
408 S.W. 2nd Ave., Rm. 403
Portland, OR 97204
(503) 223-8299 (10 A.M.–
  3 P.M.)

AIDS Hotline
P.O. Box 968
Santa Fe, NM 87504
(505) 827-3201

New Mexico Physicians for
  Human Rights
P.O. Box 1361
Espanola, NM 87532
(505) 753-2779/984-1217

AIDS Project/L.A.
937 N. Cole Ave., #3
Los Angeles, CA 90038
(213) 871-1284

SF AIDS Foundation
54 10th St.
San Francisco, CA 94104
(415) 864-4376

Diablo V. Community
  Center
1818 Colfax St.
Concord, CA 94520
(415) 827-2960

Gay & Lesbian Community
  Services of Orange
  County
12832 Garden Grove Blvd.
Garden Grove, CA 92643
(714) 534-0862

Southern California
  Physicians for Human
  Rights
7985 Santa Monica Blvd.,
  #109
Los Angeles, CA 90032
(213) 658-6261

AIDS/Kaposi's Sarcoma
  Foundation
2115 J. St., #3
Sacramento, CA 95816
(916) 448-AIDS

San Diego AIDS Project
P.O. Box 81082
San Diego, CA 92138
(619) 294-2437

San Francisco AIDS Project
P.O. Box 14227
San Francisco, CA 94114
(415) 864-4376

Shanti Project
890 Hayes St.
San Francisco, CA 94117
(415) 558-9644

Bay Area Physicians for
  Human Rights
P.O. Box 14546
San Francisco, CA 94114
(415) 558-9353 (adm.) or
  372-7321 (medical)

Berkeley Gay Men's Clinic
2339 Durrant Ave.
Berkeley, CA 94704
(415) 548-2570 or 848-9220

AIDS/KS Foundation/SC
  Co.
715 North 1st St.
San Jose, CA 95112
(408) 298-4238 (hotline, 12
  noon–9 P.M. M-F)

Colorado AIDS Project/
  GLCC
1436 Lafayette St.
Denver, CO 80218
(303) 831-6268

CENTRAL UNITED STATES

Oklahoma for Human
  Rights
4107 East 2nd Pl.
Oklahoma City, OK 74112

Health Guard Foundation
417 N.W. 9th St.
Oklahoma, OK 73102
(405) 235-5693

AIDS Committee
1627 West Rosewood
San Antonio, TX 78201
(512) 736-5216

Oaklawn AIDS Action
  Project
5811 Nash
Dallas, TX 75235
(214) 351-1502

AIDS Vol. of Cincinnati
P.O. Box 2615
Cincinnati, OH 45201
(513) 542-0493

St. Louis Task Force on
  AIDS
P.O. Box 2905
St. Louis, MO 63130
(312) 862-9800

AIDS Support Group
c/o 2309 Girard Ave. S.
Minneapolis, MN 55405

Wellness Networks, Inc.
P.O. Box 1046
Royal Oaks, MI 48068
(313) 876-3582

Howard Brown Memorial
  Clinic/AIDS Action
  Project
2676 N. Halsted St.
Chicago, IL 60614
(312) 871-5777

Kaposi's Sarcoma/AIDS
  Foundation
3317 Montrose, Box 1155
Houston, TX 77006
(713) 524-2437

National Coalition of Gay
  Sexually Transmitted
  Disease Services
P.O. Box 239
Milwaukee, WI 53201
(414) 277-7671

LGCS/MN AIDS Project
124 West Lake St.
Minneapolis, MN 55408
(612) 827-2821

AIDS Task Force
P.O. Box 190712
Dallas, TX 75219
(214) 528-4233

AIDS Task Force
1022 Barracks St.
New Orleans, LA 70116
(504) 568-9619/524-7023

APPENDIX B

Centers for Disease Control surveillance definition of the Acquired Immune Deficiency Syndrome (AIDS)

1. The presence of a reliably diagnosed disease at least moderately predictive of cellular immune deficiency.
2. The absence of an underlying cause for the immune deficiency or of any defined cause for reduced resistance to the disease.

Diseases at least moderately predictive of cellular immune deficiency:

A. **Cancers**
   1. Kaposi's sarcoma
   2. Primary Lymphoma of brain

B. **Protozoal and helminthic infections**
   1. Cryptosporidiosis, intestinal: causing diarrhea for over one month
   2. *Pneumocystis carinii* pneumonia
   3. Strongyloidosis: pneumonia, CNS infection, or disseminated infection
   4. Toxoplasmosis: pneumonia or CNS infection

C. **Fungal Infections**
   1. Aspergillosis: CNS or disseminated infection
   2. Candidiasis: esophagitis
   3. Cryptococcosis: pulmonary, CNS, or disseminated infection

D. **Bacterial infection**
   1. "Atypical" mycobacteriosis (species other than *M. tuberculosis* or *M. leprae*): disseminated infection

E. **Viral infections**
  1. Cytomegalovirus: pulmonary, gastrointestinal tract, or CNS infection
  2. Herpes simplex virus:
      a. Chronic mucocutaneous ulcers persisting more than one month, or
      b. Pulmonary, gastrointestinal tract, or disseminated infection
  3. Progressive multifocal leukoencephalopathy (presumed papovavirus)

APPENDIX C

The following refinements to the case definition of AIDS used for national reporting have been adopted by the CDC and published in the *MMWR* June 18, 1985.

1. In the absence of the opportunistic diseases required by the current case definition, any of the following diseases will be considered indicative of AIDS if the patient has a positive serologic or virologic test for HTLV-III/LAV:
   a. disseminated histoplasmosis (not confined to lungs or lymph nodes), diagnosed by culture, histology, or antigen detection;
   b. isoporiasis, causing chronic diarrhea (over 1 month), diagnosed by histology or stool microscopy;
   c. bronchial or pulmonary candidiasis, diagnosed by microscopy or by presence of characteristic white plaques grossly on the bronchial mucosa (not by culture alone);
   d. non-Hodgkin's lymphoma of high-grade pathologic type (diffuse, undifferentiated) and of B-cell or unknown immunologic phenotype, diagnosed by biopsy;

e.   histologically confirmed Kaposi's sarcoma in pa-
      tients who are 60 years old or older when diagnosed.

2. In the absence of the opportunistic diseases required by
   the current case definition, a histologically confirmed
   diagnosis of chronic lymphoid interstitial pneumonitis
   in a child (under 13 years of age) will be considered
   indicative of AIDS unless test(s) for HTLV-III/LAV are
   negative.
3. Patients who have a lymphoreticular malignancy diagnosed more than 3 months after the diagnosis of an
   opportunistic disease used as a marker for AIDS will no
   longer be excluded as AIDS cases.
4. To increase the specificity of the case definition, patients will be excluded as AIDS cases if they have a
   negative result on testing for serum antibody to HTLV-
   III/LAV, have no other type of HTLV-III/LAV test with a
   positive result, and do not have a low number of T-helper
   lymphocytes or a low ratio of T-helper to T-suppressor
   lymphocytes. In the absence of test results, patients satisfying all other criteria in the definition will continue
   to be included.

According to the CDC, this revision in the case definition will result in the reclassification of less than 1% of
cases previously reported. The number of additional new
cases reportable as a result of the revision is expected to be
small. Cases included under the revised definition will be
distinguishable from cases included under the old definition so as to provide a consistent basis for interpretation of
trends. CDC will also develop draft classifications for disease manifestations of HTLV-III/LAV infections other than
AIDS, distribute these widely for comment, and publish
the results.

GLOSSARY OF TERMS*

AIDS (acquired immunodeficiency syndrome): A disease believed to be caused by the retrovirus HTLV-III (human T-cell lymphotropic virus, type III) and characterized by a deficiency of the immune system. The primary defect in AIDS is an acquired, persistent, quantitative functional depression within the T4 subset of lymphocytes. This depression often leads to infections caused by micro-organisms that usually do not produce infections in individuals with normal immunity or to the development of a rare type of cancer (Kaposi's sarcoma) usually seen in elderly persons or in individuals who are severely immunocompromised from other causes. Other associated diseases are currently under investigation and will probably be included in the final definition of AIDS.

AIDS-related complex: A variety of chronic but nonspecific symptoms and physical findings that appear related to AIDS, which may consist of chronic generalized lymphadenopathy, recurrent fevers, weight loss, minor alterations in the immune system, and minor infections. Some persons with AIDS-related complex may develop full-blown AIDS, while in others, the condition may represent the height of clinical illness in reaction to infection with HTLV-III. AIDS-related complex is sometimes known as "pre-AIDS." (Compare "lymphadenopathy syndrome.")

Antibody: A blood protein produced by mammals in response to exposure to a specific antigen. Antibodies are a critical component of the mammalian immune system.

Antigen: A large molecule, usually a protein or carbohydrate, which when introduced into the body stimulates the production of an antibody that will react specifically with that antigen.

ARV (AIDS-related retrovirus): A retrovirus recovered

271

from an AIDS patient and believed to be the same virus as HTLV-III. (See "HTLV-III.")

B lymphocytes (or B cells): Lymphocytes that mediate humoral (e.g., antibody production) immune reactions. B lymphocytes proliferate under stimulation from factors released by T lymphocytes. (Compare "T lymphocytes.")

Cofactor: Factors or agents that are necessary or that increase the probability of the development of disease in the presence of the basic etiologic agent of that disease.

Core proteins: Proteins that make up the internal structure or core of a virus. (Compare "envelope proteins.")

Cytopathic: Pertaining to or characterized by abnormal changes in cells.

Envelope proteins: Proteins that comprise the envelope or surface of a virus. (Compare "core proteins.")

Enzyme: Any of a group of catalytic proteins that are produced by living cells and that mediate and promote the chemical processes of life without themselves being altered or destroyed.

Epidemiologic studies: Studies concerned with the relationships of various factors determining the frequency and distribution of specific diseases in a human community.

Etiologic agent: Causative agent.

Factor VIII: A naturally occurring protein in plasma that aids in the coagulation of blood. A congenital deficiency of Factor VIII results in the bleeding disorder known as hemophilia A.

Factor VIII concentrate: A concentrated preparation of Factor VIII that is used in the treatment of individuals with hemophilia A.

Gene: The basic unit of heredity; an ordered sequence of nucleotide bases, comprising a segment of DNA. A gene contains the sequence of DNA that encodes for the synthesis of one polypeptide chain (protein).

Genome: The genetic endowment of an organism.

Hemophilia: A rare, hereditary bleeding disorder caused

by a deficiency in the ability to synthesize one or more of the blood coagulation proteins, e.g., Factor VIII (hemophilia A) or Factor IX (hemophilia B).

Hepatitis: Inflammation of the liver; may be due to many causes, including viruses, several of which are transmissible through blood transfusions.

HPA-23 (heteropolytungstate): A drug that has been shown to inhibit the reverse transcriptase enzyme of murine (mouse) retrovirus in vitro and in vivo, and which has been shown in early clinical trials to inhibit HTLV-III replication in humans, but which has not eradicated the virus. (Compare "ribavirin" and "suramin.")

HTLV-III (human T-cell lymphotropic virus, type III): A newly discovered retrovirus that is believed to be the basic cause of AIDS. The target organ of HTLV-III is the T4 subset of T lymphocytes, which are the master regulators of the immune system. HTLV-III is used to refer to the various isolates (e.g., LAV, ARV) that have been associated with AIDS.

Immune: Being highly resistant to a disease because of the formation of humoral antibodies or the development of cellular immunity, or both, or as a result of some other mechanism (e.g., interferon activity in viral infections).

Interferon: A class of glycoproteins (proteins with carbohydrates attached at specific locations) important in immune function and thought to inhibit viral infections.

In vitro: Literally, "in glass"; pertaining to a biological reaction taking place in an artificial apparatus; often used in reference to the growth of cells from multicellular organisms under cell culture conditions.

In vivo: Literally, "in the living"; pertaining to a biological reaction taking place in a living organism.

Kaposi's sarcoma: A multifocal, spreading cancer of connective tissue, principally involving the skin; it usually begins on the toes or the feet as reddish blue or brownish soft nodules and tumors.

LAV (lymphadenopathy-associated virus): A retrovirus recovered from a person with lymphadenopathy (enlarged lymph nodes) who was also in a group at high risk for AIDS, and now believed to be the same virus as HTLV-III. (See 'HTLV-III.")

Lymphadenopathy: Enlargement of the lymph nodes.

Lymphadenopathy syndrome (LAS): A condition which is characterized by persistent, generalized, enlarged lymph nodes, sometimes with signs of minor illness such as fever and weight loss, which apparently represents a milder reaction to infection with HTLV-III than full-blown AIDS. Some patients with LAS have gone on to develop full-blown AIDS, while in others, LAS may represent the height of clinical illness in reaction to infection with HTLV-III. LAS is also known as "generalized lymphadenopathy syndrome." (Compare "AIDS-related complex.")

Lymphocytes: Specialized white blood cells involved in the immune response. (See also "B lymphocytes" and "T lymphocytes.")

Opportunistic infection: A disease or infection caused by a micro-organism that does not ordinarily cause disease but which, under certain conditions (e.g., impaired immune responses), becomes pathologic.

Pneumocystis carinii pneumonia: A type of pneumonia primarily found in infants and now commonly occurring in patients with AIDS.

Provirus: The genome of an animal virus integrated into the chromosome of the host cell, and thereby replicated in all of the host's daughter cells.

Recombinant DNA techniques: Techniques that allow specific segments of DNA to be isolated and inserted into a bacterium or other host (e.g., yeast, mammalian cells) in a form that will allow the DNA segment to be replicated and expressed as the cellular host multiplies. The DNA segment is said to be "cloned" because it exists free of the rest of DNA of the organism from which it was derived.

Retroviruses: Viruses that contain RNA, not DNA, and that produce a DNA analog of their RNA through the production of an enzyme known as "reverse transcriptase." The resulting DNA is incorporated in the genetic structure of the invaded cell in a form referred to as the "provirus." (See also "provirus" and "viruses.")

Ribavirin: A drug thath has been shown to protect T4 cells against infection by HTLV-III in vitro, and which is being tested in AIDS patients. (Compare "suramin" and "HPA-23.")

Serum: The clear portion of any animal liquid separated from its more solid elements, especially the clear liquid (blood serum) which separates in the clotting of blood.

Suramin: A drug that has been shown to protect T4 cells against infection by HTLV-III in vitro, and which is being tested in AIDS patients. (Compare "ribavirin" and HPA-23.")

T-cell growth factor (TCGF, also known as interleukin-2): A glycoprotein that is released by T lymphocytes on stimulation with antigens and which functions as a T-cell growth factor by inducing proliferation of activated T cells. (See also "T lymphocytes.")

T lymphocytes (or T cells): Lymphocytes that mature in the thymus and which mediate cellular immune reactions. T lymphocytes also release factors that induce proliferation of T lymphocytes and B lymphocytes. (Compare "B lymphocytes.")

Tropism: An innate tendency to react in a definite manner to stimuli.

Vaccine: A preparation of killed organisms, living attenuated organisms, living fully virulent organisms or parts of micro-organisms, that is administered to produce or artificially increase immunity to a particular disease.

Viruses: Any of a large group of submicroscopic agents capable of infecting plants, animals, and bacteria and characterized by a total dependence on living cells for reproduction and by a lack of independent metabolism.

*Reprinted—*Review of the Public Health Service's Response to AIDS* (Washington, DC: U.S. Congress, Office of Technology Assessment, OTA-TM-H-24, February 1985).

Index